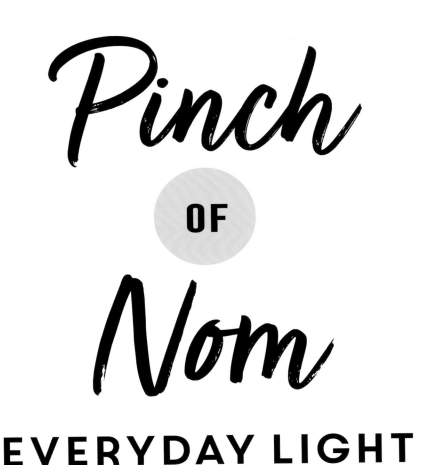

Pinch

OF

Nom

EVERYDAY LIGHT

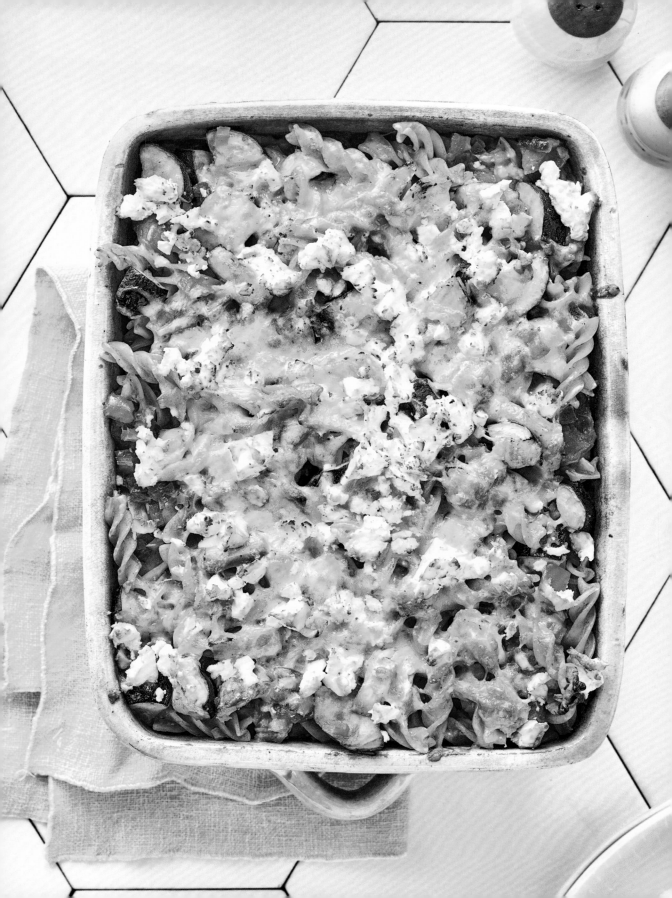

ZA'ATAR CHICKEN is so *tasty* and *filling!*

JUDITH

Everyone in my house *loves* HASH BROWN BREAKFAST BAKE

KEZ

SLOPPY DOGS: #PINCHOFNOMNOMNOM

ANITA

MY HUSBAND INHALED *the* CHIPOTLE PORK BURGERS!

CHARLEE

GARLIC AND LIME BALTI *is absolutely gorgeous!*

CHELSEA

The QUESADILLA *is* UTTERLY DELICIOUS

JACKIE

LEMON PEPPER CHICKEN TAGLIATELLE was *demolished* with praise and requests to make again

ANITA

TANDOORI SALMON WITH MANGO SALSA will *definitely* be a regular dish in our house

JIM

The VEGETABLE PARMESAN CHIPS are so *tasty* and *crispy!*

JUDITH

CHICKEN DOPIAZA is very *tasty* and incredibly simple to make.

CATHY

KATE ALLINSON & KAY FEATHERSTONE

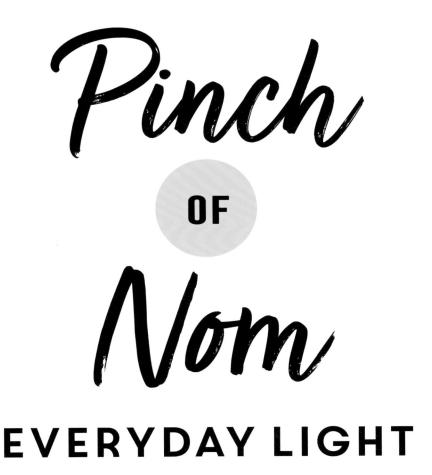

Pinch

OF

Nom

EVERYDAY LIGHT

100 TASTY, SLIMMING RECIPES
ALL UNDER 400 CALORIES

bluebird
books for life

First published 2019 by Bluebird
an imprint of Pan Macmillan
The Smithson, 6 Briset Street, London EC1M 5NR

Associated companies throughout the world
www.panmacmillan.com

ISBN 978-1-5290-2640-5

5 7 9 8 6 4
A CIP catalogue record for this book is available from the British Library.
Printed and bound in Italy.

Publisher Carole Tonkinson
Managing Editor Martha Burley
Senior Production Controller Sarah Badhan
Art Direction and Design Emma Wells, Nic&Lou
Illustration Shutterstock / Emma Wells
Food Styling Kate Wesson
Prop Styling Cynthia Blackett

Visit www.panmacmillan.com to read more about all our books
and to buy them. You will also find features, author interviews and
news of any author events, and you can sign up for e-newsletters
so that you're always first to hear about our new releases.

Contents

WELCOME

to

Pinch

OF

Nom

EVERYDAY LIGHT!

Wow! Our second book! We still can't believe how much you guys liked the first. We were overwhelmed by all your support and by how much you loved making the recipes. We enjoyed watching post after post in our Facebook group of all the recipes being made. That's what it's all about for us – getting people back into the kitchen and cooking for all the family, while also giving you healthy, calorie-friendly swaps. So . . . we're back again with this: the Everyday Light book.

SO WHAT DOES 'EVERYDAY LIGHT' MEAN?

Well, the simple answer is that all of the meals in this book come in under 400 calories. But we've made sure to use the right ingredients so you're still getting decent portions! We don't create recipes where you only got a teaspoon of food – we want to give you the same hearty Pinch of Nom food you've come to know and love. All of these dishes are either complete meals, or we have suggested an accompaniment that will still bring the dish under 400 calories (you can also refer to our list of accompaniments and calorie counts on page 265). If you're following the major diet plans in the UK, all of the recipes can be enjoyed without counting any values, aside from any fibre and dairy allowances. We've made sure that all of the recipes work on the major diet plans, as well as for calorie-counting.

Everyday Light recipes have been requested by the community so many times, we've lost count! So we're delighted to finally be able to put all these together for you in this beautiful book.

The majority of these recipes are packed with vegetables and protein – perfect for keeping meals lean, while making sure you're full until your next meal. Of course, for a few extra calories, we have some sides and snacks – but, if you're calorie-counting, keep an eye on your main meal calories before adding on the sides.

We can hear you thinking 'meat and veg' and rolling your eyes. But we promise, these are still the Pinch of Nom meals you know and love – Fish and Chips (see page 48), Pizza-loaded Fries (see page 74), Sloppy Dogs (see page 65), and Firecracker Prawns (see page 72), to name but a few. We've used our tried and tested way of seasoning, flavouring and spicing the meals so you won't find bland meat with a side salad – that's not what we're about!

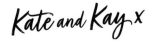

THE FOOD

MADE WITH LOVE

As a classically trained chef, Kate has always looked at well-known recipes and dishes, then worked out how to improve or recreate them. That is still the case and it's how the Pinch of Nom recipes are formed. She and her small team come up with the best ideas for recipes, then get into the kitchen and throw around ingredients until they find the right balance.

FAST METHODS *and* FAMILIAR INGREDIENTS

You can prepare most of the recipes in this book in under 30 minutes. It was important to the Pinch of Nom team that the recipes were easily accessible and featured ingredients that home cooks will use time and again to save on cost. Ingredients that are less familiar are only used when they add a unique touch to the dish — and we make sure they are used more than once so you'll never have ingredients gathering dust.

SIMPLE METHODS

We've also made sure that the recipes work for any cooking ability. We didn't want gourmet chefs as our taste testers — or even have a requirement that people needed to be able to cook. We wanted a subsection of the general public to attempt these recipes and see how they got on. Based on their feedback, we're confident that even the novice cook can tackle these recipes and end up with a decent meal without spending hours in the kitchen.

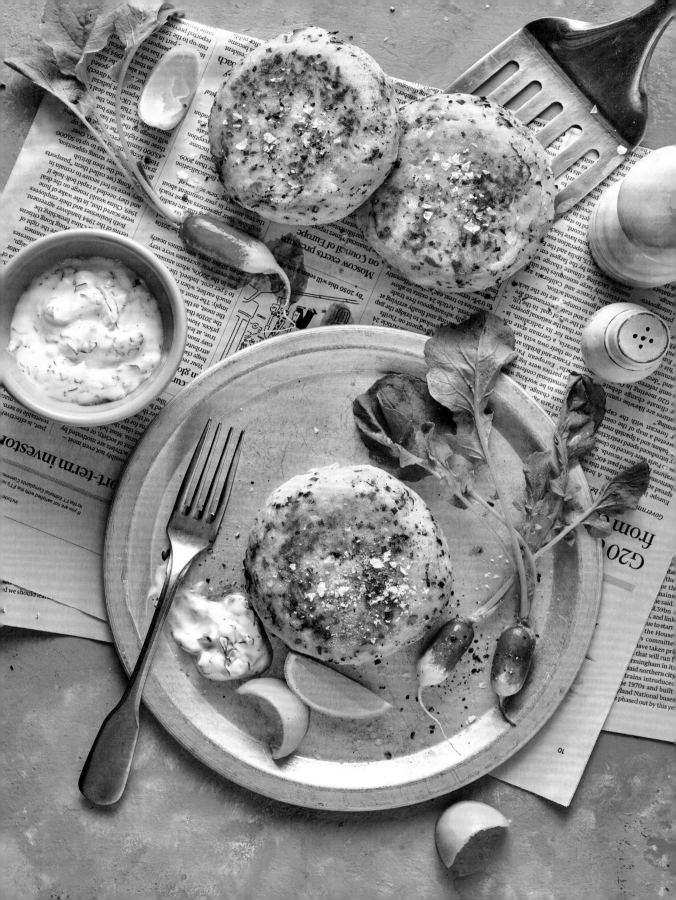

BATCH COOK

We've grouped our favourite batch-cooking recipes together in their own chapter, because batch-cooking ideas are often requested by our community. As you can see, these recipes have their own specific guidelines, but there are also plenty of other recipes in the book that you can batch cook with a few tweaks. Some general notes to think about when batch cooking are below. It's always important to store food safely, so we have included the latest NHS food-safety guidelines (correct at the time of writing).

- **Divide the food into individual portions** to refrigerate or freeze. This means you can just reheat one portion, or four portions, or six etc. without needing to chisel portions off of one big frozen block! It will also ensure they cool and freeze (and defrost) quicker.

- **Make sure you've got enough space** in your fridge or freezer for your meals before you get cooking!

- **Use refrigerated foods within 2 days**.

- **When freezing food**, make sure you use airtight containers or freezer bags that are suitable for the freezer. Invest in some decent, freezer- and microwave-proof storage containers. If not, your containers may crack or melt, which is not what you need when you want a quick meal you've spent time batch cooking. Make sure your containers are sealed properly to avoid 'freezer burn', which is when the food has been damaged by oxidization from air getting inside.

- **Always label food**. Use freezer-proof stickers to label your dish, adding the date when you made it. Nobody wants mystery food in the freezer, and it's likely it will end up going to waste. Meals can be frozen for around 3–6 months. Up to 3 months is ideal and beyond 6 months is still safe, but the food may not taste as good.

- **Always make sure food is defrosted thoroughly before reheating it**, either in the fridge or microwave.

- **Only reheat food once**.

- **When food has defrosted** completely, it should be reheated and eaten within 24 hours, so only defrost what you need. NHS guidelines state you should reheat food until it reaches 70°C/130°F and holds that temperature for 2 minutes. Make sure it is piping hot all the way through. Stir during reheating to ensure this.

- **You may freeze the sauce or meat** for some recipes, but need to cook rice, pasta or other accompaniments at the time you want to eat as they either cannot be reheated, or they're a lot nicer cooked fresh. Keep an eye out for the freezer instructions throughout the book for further details on each recipe.

- **If you are batch-cooking rice**, it's important you store it correctly before you reheat it. You should cool it as quickly as possible, ideally within 1 hour. (With other foods this could be up to 2 hours.) You can put rice in a wide, shallow container, which will help it cool quicker due to the larger surface area. There is a risk of bacteria growing the longer it is left at room temperature. Cooked rice should only be kept in the fridge for 1 day before reheating. When you reheat rice, make sure it is piping hot all the way through. Never reheat rice more than once.

How our RECIPES WORK

The recipes in this book include lots of guidance to make life easy for you. We have worked with a registered nutritionist, but all of these calculations and dietary indicators are only for guidance and are not to be taken as complete fact — make sure you also check the ingredients and food labels yourself.

KCALS PER SERVING

All of our recipes have been worked out as complete meals, using standardized portion sizes for any accompaniments as advised by the British Nutrition Foundation.

GLUTEN FREE

We have marked gluten-free recipes with an icon (see right). We have also made suggestions for the use of gluten-free variants of common ingredients, such as stock cubes and Worcestershire sauce. Please check the labelling to ensure the product you buy is a gluten-free variant.

VEGETARIAN

Nearly half of the recipes in this book are veggie and you can easily make more recipes meat-free by swapping out non-veggie ingredients such as Parmesan and Worcestershire sauce. Look out for our Make it Veggie boxes that offer extra guidance.

OUR RECIPE ICONS

V   Suitable for vegetarians

F   Suitable for freezing
For all freezer-friendly recipes, we recommend defrosting completely before heating until piping hot.

GF   Suitable for those following a gluten-free diet

TASTE TESTED

A group of two hundred Pinch of Nom fans have been huddled together on a secret Facebook group to test these recipes. Each recipe has been tested by twenty people, all submitting feedback and suggestions for development to ensure that we're not the only ones who love the food in the book.

This process has been essential in the creation of this book and we want to extend a huge thank you to these members for their invaluable input. (You can find their names in the back of the book.)

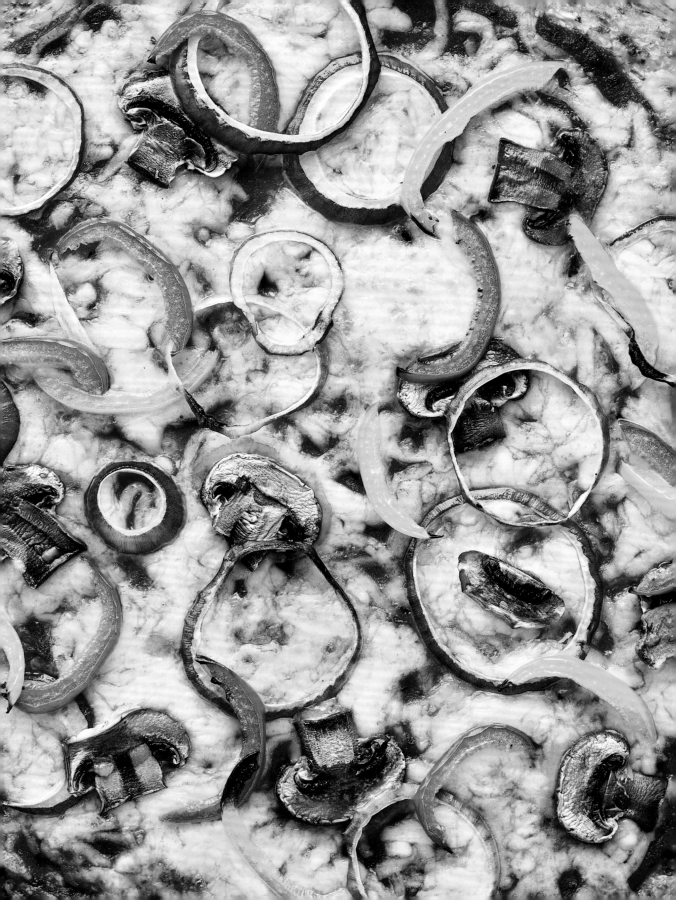

KEY INGREDIENTS

PROTEIN

Lean meats are a great source of protein, providing essential nutrients and fantastic filling power. In all recipes with meat as an ingredient, make sure you use the leanest cuts and trim off all visible fat. Fish is another great source of protein and is naturally low in fat. One of our favourite phrases is: 'if it swims, it slims'! Fish provides nutrients that the body struggles to produce naturally, making it perfect for some of Pinch of Nom's super-slimming recipes. Just under half of the recipes in this book are veggie, but you can always use vegetarian protein options instead of meat in our recipes (though this will affect the calorie count).

STOCKS and SAUCES

One of Pinch of Nom's favourite ingredients is the lowly stock pot. It adds instant flavour and is so versatile. We use various flavoured pots throughout this book, but they are all interchangeable. Wine stock pots are a genius invention – flavour without the calories! We also love soy, fish and Worcestershire sauces for big splashes of flavour. It is worth noting that these ingredients are often high in salt, so swap with reduced-salt varieties if you prefer.

TINS and FROZEN FOODS

Don't be afraid to bulk-buy some of those tinned essentials! Beans, tomatoes, sweetcorn . . . You'll find you can add many of these ingredients to Pinch of Nom stews and salads. They keep the cost of dishes down and, compared to fresh, it makes little or no difference to the flavour. Similarly, frozen veggies bulk out dishes and are great low-cost alternatives for recipes like stews, where fresh options aren't necessarily required.

LOW-FAT DAIRY

Swapping in clever alternatives for high-fat dairy products can instantly make a dish healthier. We often substitute low-fat soft cheese or yoghurt for higher-fat ingredients.

LOW-CALORIE SPRAY

One of the best ways to cut down on cooking with oils and fats is to use a low-calorie cooking spray. It makes little difference to the way that most ingredients are cooked, but it has a huge impact on the calories because you need so much less than you would when pouring oil into a pan. You can also use olive oil spray – just be careful how much you're spraying to save calories.

HERBS *and* SPICES

Pinch of Nom love a bit of spice! When you're changing ingredients for lower fat/sugar/calorie versions, one of the best ways to keep your food interesting is to season it well with herbs and spices. In particular, mixed spice blends are perfect for lots of recipes in this book. Don't be shy with spices – not all of them burn your mouth off! We use garlic granules in a lot of our recipes because they are a convenient and cheaper alternative to fresh garlic and in slow cooks and stews, for example, you won't be able to tell the difference.

EGGS

Protein-rich, filling, tasty and versatile, eggs are the ultimate slimming yet satisfying ingredient. Start your day with a filling, protein-rich Egg-in-the-hole Breakfast Bagel (see page 29) or try them on top of a comforting, sustaining Ramen Bowl (see page 168). You'll always want a box in the house.

VINEGARS

When you remove fat from a recipe, flavours can dwindle. Carefully adding vinegar can bring rich, deep balance to flavours. Some people use spices for this purpose, but acidity levels are also really important.

TORTILLA WRAPS

Pinch of Nom recipes are synonymous with creating magic with wraps! You'll be surprised at the dishes you can make using a lowly wrap – you can even use it in place of pastry (see our Plait recipe, page 100). Wholewheat or wholegrain wraps provide fibre and filling power, too.

BREAD

We use gluten-free rolls in some of our recipes. Generally lower in calories, they have a high fibre-density, which is a perfect way to balance a low-calorie diet. We also use some wholemeal bread – another great source of fibre providing that all-important filling power. Try it broken down into breadcrumbs to make coatings for meat (see Popcorn Chicken, page 56).

LEMONS *and* LIMES

Citrus fruits pack a punch when it comes to flavour. They're perfect for adding to recipes that need an extra bit of 'zing'.

PULSES, RICE *and* BEANS

High in both protein and fibre, tins of beans and pulses are perfect cupboard staples. Rice is really satisfying and, when flavoured with spices and/or seasoning, it's a great accompaniment to many of our recipes.

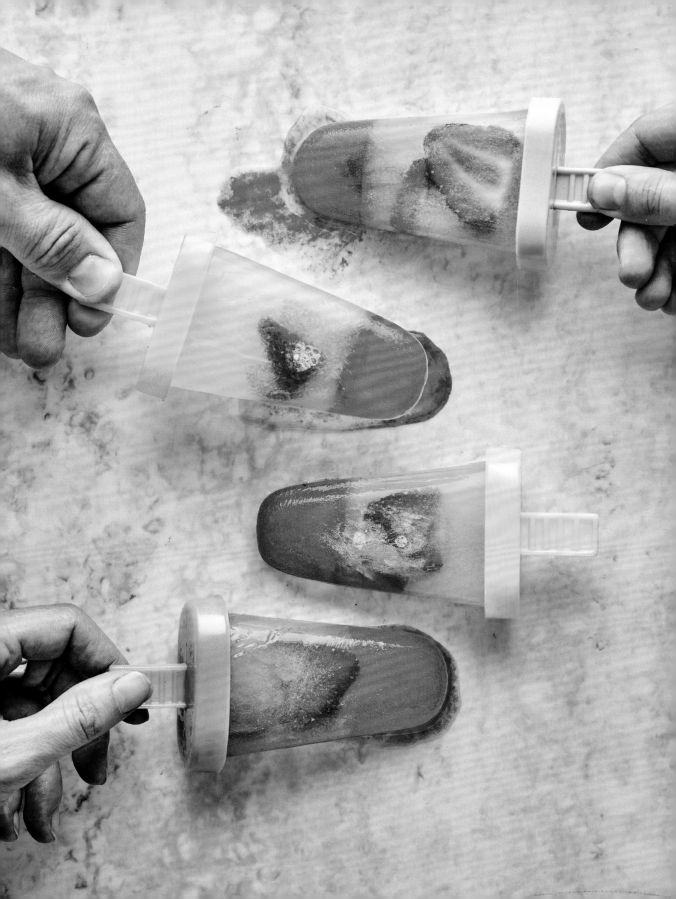

DELICIOUS · FOOD ·

Hassle-free Slimming

ESSENTIAL KIT

NON-STICK PANS

If there's one bit of kit that we'd recommend more than any other, it's a decent set of non-stick pans. The better the non-stick quality of your pans, the less cooking oils and fats you will need to avoid food sticking to your pan and burning. Keep your pans in good health, too – clean them properly and gently with soapy water.

MEASURING SPOONS

Want to make sure you're not putting a tablespoon of chilli powder in your dish, rather than half a teaspoon? This is one of the most helpful items of kitchenware you'll ever own. Especially vital if you've ever made the aforementioned mistake, as we have never done. Never.

TUPPERWARE *and* PLASTIC TUBS

Most of the Pinch of Nom recipes in this book are freezable and ideal for batch cooking (see our mini guide on pages 10–11). Planning ahead is so much easier when you can cook ahead too. So invest in some decent freezer-proof tubs for storage.

FOOD PROCESSOR / BLENDER / STICK BLENDER

Many of our recipes involve making delicious, flavourful sauces from scratch, so a decent blender or food processor is a godsend! You can also use a stick blender on most occasions, if you're looking for something a bit cheaper or more compact.

FINE GRATER

Using a fine grater is one of those surprising revelations. You won't believe the difference in grating cheese with a fine grater versus a standard grater. Around 45g of cheese, for example, can easily cover an oven dish when using a fine grater. It's much easier to keep calories down and make your cheese go much further!

OVEN TRAYS

Used in a high percentage of Pinch of Nom dishes, oven trays are an essential bit of kit – keep them in good condition for longer by using disposable baking paper or foil to line them before cooking.

KNIFE SHARPENER

There is nothing worse than trying to chop a butternut squash up with a spoon. So why would you recreate the experience with your knives? Keep those babies sharp! It will save you so much time and effort.

SPATULA

This is an essential bit of kit. If you don't own one, you really should! You'll be surprised how indispensable it will become.

POTATO MASHER

Used in a variety of recipes, you'll need a decent masher to ensure you're not straining muscles every time you want a bit of mash. We've recently discovered masher attachments on stick blenders and we are OBSESSED! We recommend using one for achieving the silkiest and smoothest mash ever.

SLOW COOKER and PRESSURE COOKER

These are more of an optional favourite than essential, but we absolutely love them. Electric pressure cookers and slow cookers are perfect for quick family meals that are made without having to stand over a cooker. Also, don't be fooled into thinking that you have to buy expensive cuts of meat for the best results. Cheaper cuts of meat often end up being tastier and more tender when slow or pressure cooking, which is a bonus for flavour and for your wallet! Try our winning Cherry Cola Pulled Pork (page 156) or the Beef and Sweet Potato Stew (page 154).

WAFFLE MAKER

Not every kitchen has one, but a good waffle maker can be life-changing. We're not even exaggerating! You can use it for making sweet or savoury waffles for breakfast, dessert and everything in between. They're also relatively cheap gadgets and turn out the perfect waffle every time.

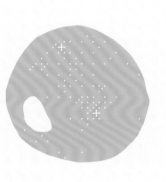

Breakfast

MONTE CRISTO SANDWICH

🕐 **5 MINS** | 🍲 **4 MINS** | ✕ **SERVES 1**

This sandwich is a variation on the classic croque monsieur. A fried ham-and-cheese sandwich doesn't sound like something you can enjoy while slimming, but by measuring your cheese and cooking with low-calorie cooking spray you can recreate the amazing flavours but keep the calories low.

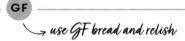

GF

↳ *use GF bread and relish*

PER SERVING:
379 KCAL
28G CARBS

2 slices of wholemeal bread
20g reduced-fat Cheddar
2 slices of lean ham (about 50g)
½ spring onion, trimmed and
   thinly sliced
1 cherry tomato, thinly sliced
3 spinach leaves, roughly chopped
1 small egg
1 tsp fat-free natural yoghurt
½ tsp Worcestershire sauce
   or Henderson's relish
¼ tsp mustard powder
sea salt and freshly ground
   black pepper
low-calorie cooking spray

Cut the crusts off the slices of bread. Grate the cheese with a fine grater and sprinkle half of it onto one slice of the bread. Layer the ham, spring onion, tomato slices and spinach on top. Sprinkle over the other half of the cheese and place the second piece of bread on top. Press down on the sandwich to flatten it.

In a shallow bowl, beat the egg with the natural yoghurt and Worcestershire sauce. Season the egg with mustard powder, salt and pepper. Dip the sandwich in the egg, turning it over to make sure both sides of the bread have been soaked well.

Liberally spray a non-stick frying pan with low-calorie cooking spray and turn the heat up to medium. When the pan is hot and the cooking spray is bubbling, place the sandwich in the pan.

Cook for 1–2 minutes. Spray the top side of the sandwich with low-calorie cooking spray before flipping it over, then cook for another 1–2 minutes. The sandwich is ready when it looks golden and toasted, and the cheese has melted.

Slice the sandwich in half with a sharp knife and serve hot.

Tip

Use the strongest flavour reduced-fat Cheddar you can find – there's no place for mild cheese in this sandwich!

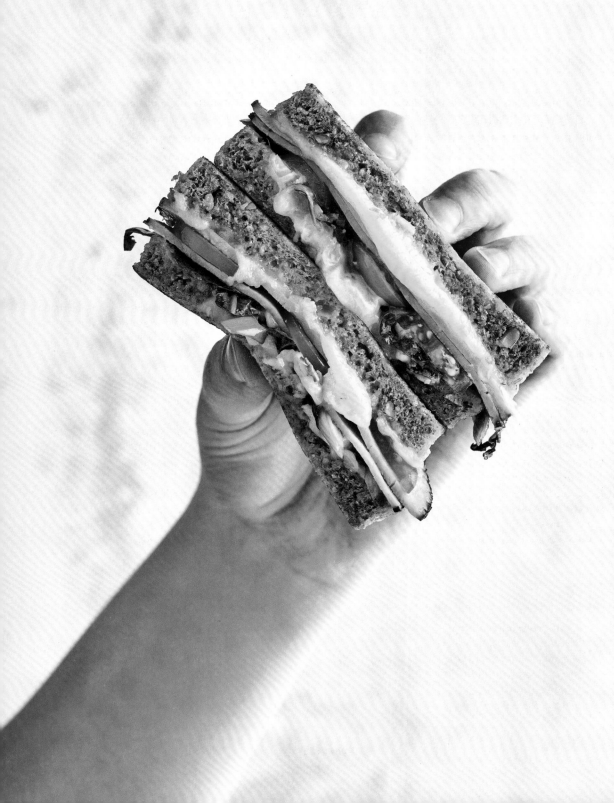

BREAKFAST
BANANA SPLIT

🕐 **5 MINS** | 🍲 **NO COOK** | ✕ **SERVES 2**

One of Kate's favourite desserts as a child was a banana split; the more cream, the better! This simple twist of using flavoured yoghurt makes it much friendlier to the waistline while making it perfect for a quick breakfast without the need to cook. Topped off with cherries, strawberries and flaked almonds, this feels like such an indulgence for just 232 calories.

PER SERVING:
232 KCAL
27G CARBS

2 bananas (about 160g each)
200g fat-free Greek yoghurt
1 tbsp granulated sweetener
   tsp vanilla extract
10 blueberries
4 strawberries
25g flaked almonds (toast them if you wish)
2 fresh cherries

Peel the bananas and slice them in half lengthways. Arrange them on two plates.

Mix the Greek yoghurt, sweetener and vanilla extract together. Thinly slice the blueberries and strawberries, reserving two strawberry halves for garnish. Stir the sliced berries into the yoghurt.

Spoon the yoghurt mix onto the middle of the bananas. Sprinkle the flaked almonds on top and decorate with a fresh cherry and the reserved halved strawberries.

Tip

Don't like nuts? You could use a sprinkling of your favourite cereal or muesli in this recipe instead.

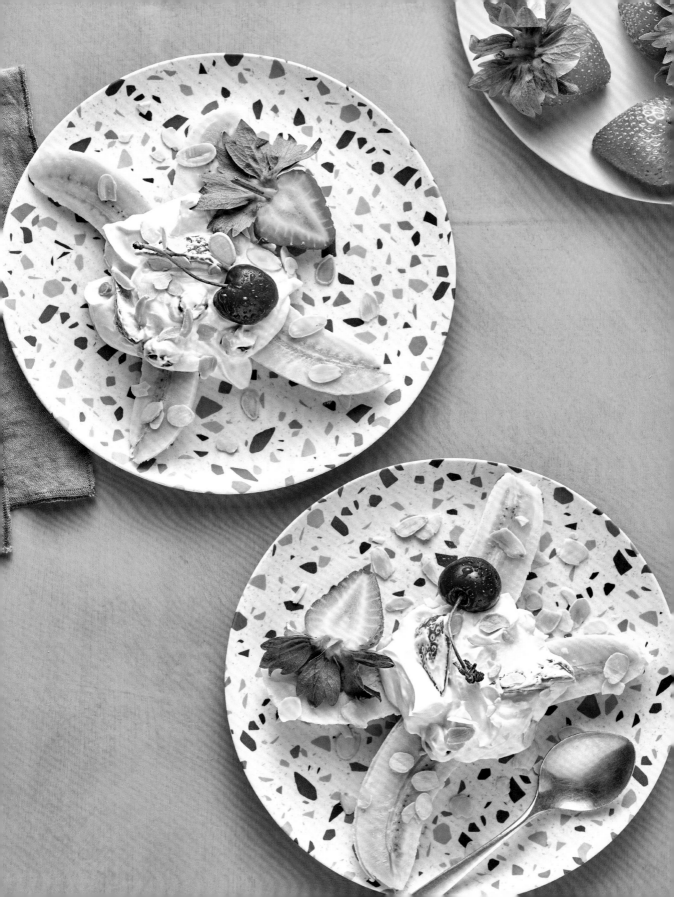

CHEESY LEEKS
on TOAST

🕐 **5 MINS** | 🍲 **15 MINS** | 🍴 **SERVES 2**

Sometimes, you just need a quick fix for a tasty brekkie in a flash. You might think that a creamy cheese sauce would be off the menu, but by using a few clever ingredient swaps, you will have plenty of calories to play with! Using a strong-tasting hard cheese alongside a little Cheddar, you can pack in the cheese flavour without needing to use mountains of the stuff. It will satisfy even the greatest cheese-lover.

use a veggie hard cheese ↙   ↘ *use GF bread*

PER SERVING:
335 KCAL
35G CARBS

1 large leek, trimmed, washed and thinly sliced
low-calorie cooking spray
1 tbsp water
pinch of sea salt
30g Italian hard cheese
20g reduced-fat Cheddar cheese
175ml skimmed milk
½ tsp mustard powder
½ tsp xanthan gum
4 small slices of wholemeal bread
mustard, to serve (optional)

Spray a small saucepan with low-calorie cooking spray and add the sliced leek with the tablespoon of water and pinch of salt. Cook the leeks for 5–7 minutes until softened and tender.

Meanwhile, finely grate the hard cheese and reduced-fat Cheddar cheese.

Once the leeks are cooked, add the milk and mustard powder to the saucepan. Bring to the boil. Take off the heat and whisk in the xanthan gum. The sauce should thicken immediately.

Return the saucepan to a low heat and add most of the cheese, reserving a little to sprinkle on later. Stir well for about 2 minutes, until the cheese is melted. The cheesy leeks should be like a thick custard – if you need to, add a little more xanthan gum, remembering that a little goes a long way.

Turn on the grill and toast the bread lightly on both sides. Once toasted, top with the cheesy leeks and sprinkle over the remaining cheese. Pop back under the grill for 3–4 minutes until bubbling and golden and serve immediately, with a little mustard (if desired).

Tip
Xanthan gum acts as an ingenious binding agent. It is gluten-free, so you'll find it in the 'free-from' supermarket aisles.

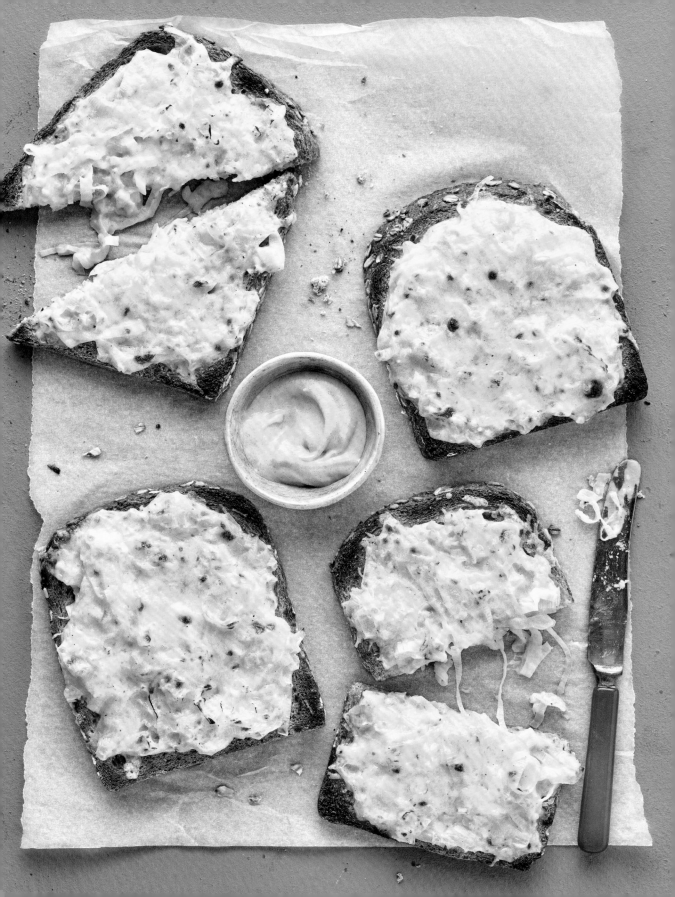

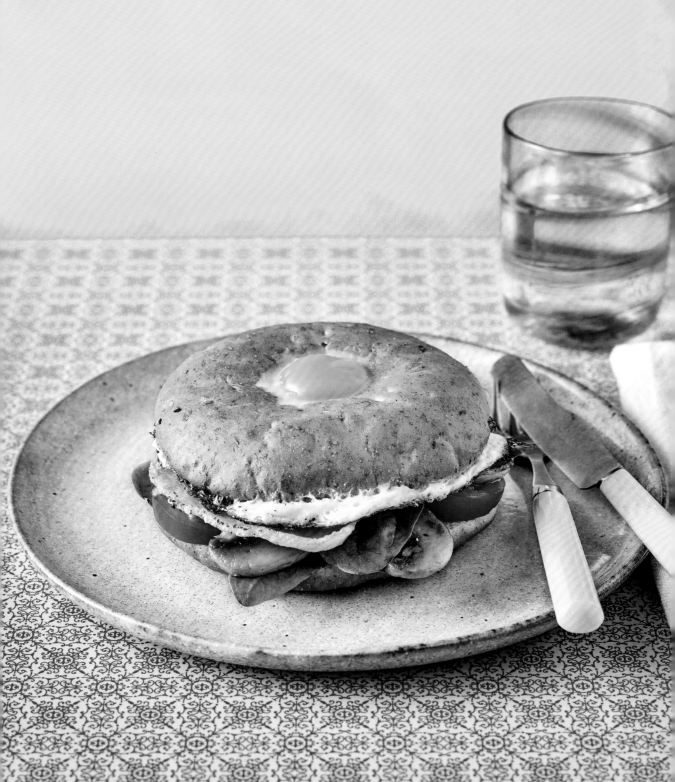

EGG-*in-the*-HOLE
BREAKFAST BAGEL

🕐 **5 MINS** | 🍲 **8–12 MINS** | ✕ **SERVES 1**

Wholemeal bagel thins are the key to keeping this dish light enough for an everyday breakfast. They have far fewer calories than their traditional counterparts, which are well known for being high in calories. The thins still give that amazing 'bagelicious' taste – and the hole in the middle? We want more! We add an egg to make it even more filling and tasty. You may need a knife and fork to eat this one if you like your yolk runny!

PER SERVING:
325 KCAL
27G CARBS

low-calorie cooking spray
2 bacon medallions
1 mushroom, sliced
sea salt and freshly ground
   black pepper
1 egg
1 wholemeal bagel thin
a few spinach leaves
2 cherry tomatoes, sliced

Spray a large frying pan with low-calorie cooking spray and set on a medium heat. Place the bacon medallions and the sliced mushroom around the edge of the pan. Season the mushroom with salt and pepper.

Separate the egg. Pour the egg white into the centre of the pan and place the top half of the bagel thin on top. Pour the egg yolk into the centre hole of the bagel in the pan. After a couple of minutes, flip the bacon and mushrooms and place a lid over the pan.

When the egg is done to your liking (for a runny yolk it will take around 8 minutes, firmer will take around 12 minutes), take the pan off the heat.

Assemble the bagel on a plate using the bottom of the bagel thin, spinach, mushroom, bacon and tomatoes and place the egg-topped bagel half on top. Season the egg with salt and pepper and serve.

MAKE *it* VEGGIE

Omit the bacon and add another sliced mushroom.

SAUSAGE *and* EGG ENGLISH MUFFIN

🕐 **5 MINS** | 🍲 **10 MINS** | ✕ **SERVES 4**

Who needs the drive-through when you can make these delicious Sausage and Egg English Muffins at home? By using lean pork mince to create your own sausage patties you can indulge in this classic breakfast sandwich for far fewer calories and fat than the takeaway version, but still have the feeling of indulgence. Yes!

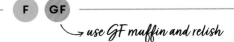

F GF

↳ *use GF muffin and relish*

PER SERVING:
377 KCAL
26G CARBS

4 wholemeal English muffins,
  sliced in half (we like Asda
  wholemeal muffins)
low-calorie cooking spray
4 small eggs
4 lighter burger cheese slices

FOR THE SAUSAGE PATTIES
400g 5%-fat pork mince
¼ tsp dried parsley
¼ tsp garlic granules
¼ tsp dried sage
½ tsp Worcestershire sauce
  or Henderson's relish
sea salt and freshly ground
  black pepper

Mix the patty ingredients together in a bowl. Knead the mince for a smoother texture. Split the mix into eight equal-sized balls. Flatten each ball and shape into a patty until you have eight thin burgers a little wider than your muffins. (You could do this the night before and keep them chilled, separated by greaseproof paper, ready for frying in the morning.)

Spray a non-stick frying pan with low-calorie cooking spray and place over a medium heat. Cook the patties for 4 minutes on each side. When done, they will have coloured on the outside and be cooked through. Place the patties on a plate under some foil to keep warm. (At this point, if you want to keep the patties for another day, cool and freeze, remembering to defrost them thoroughly before frying them.)

Lightly toast the muffins in the toaster or under the grill.

Spray the pan with some more low-calorie cooking spray and fry your eggs for 3 minutes over a medium heat with the lid on (use an egg ring or a 1-egg pan to give them a uniform shape, if you wish). When ready, the white will be opaque and the yolk will be slightly set on top. Cook for 1 minute longer if you like your yolks fully set. Season the eggs with salt and pepper.

Assemble each muffin with two sausage patties, a slice of cheese and an egg, and serve.

MAKE *it* VEGGIE

Swap the sausage patties for quorn sausage patties.

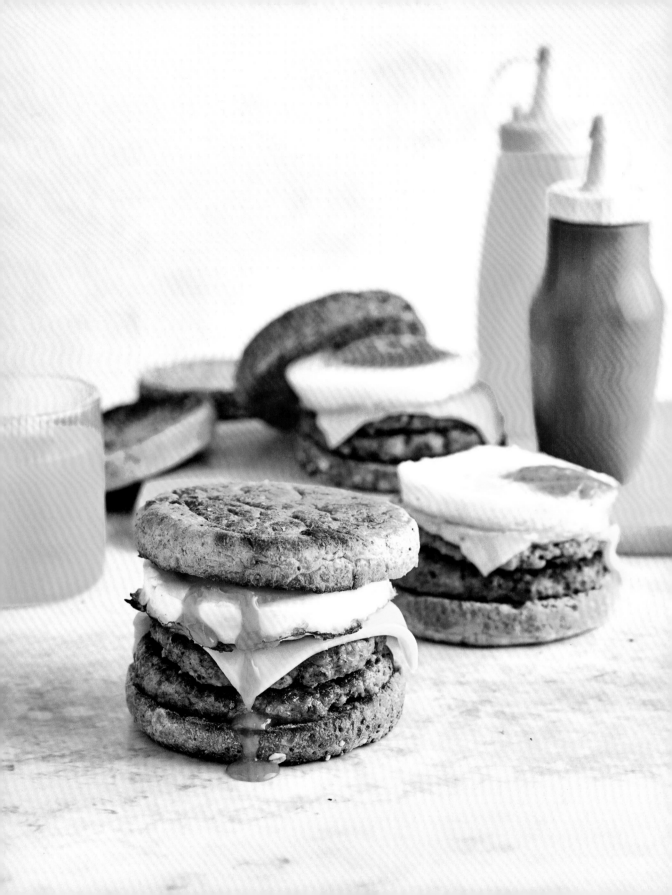

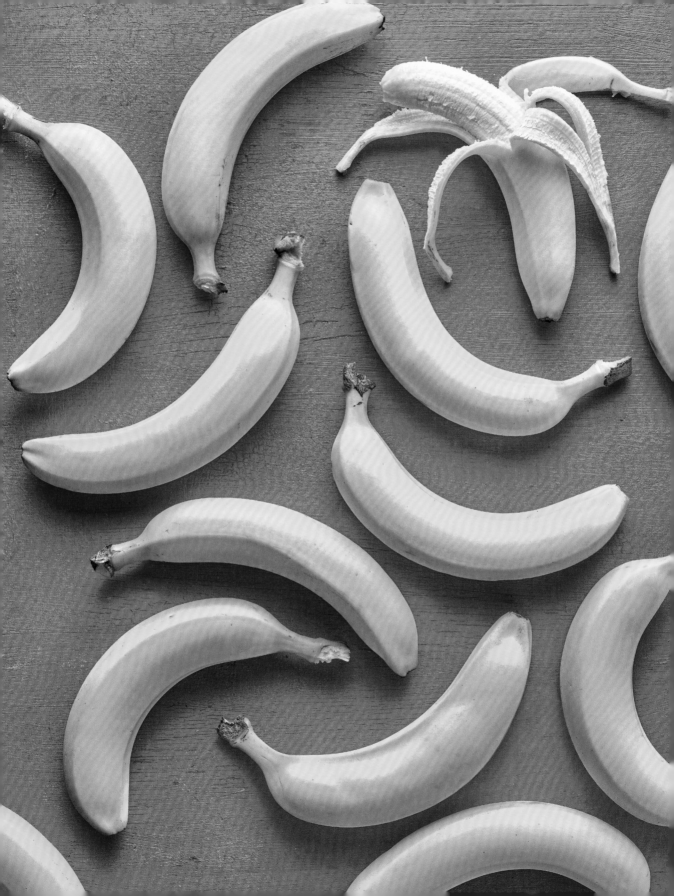

The

GIANT

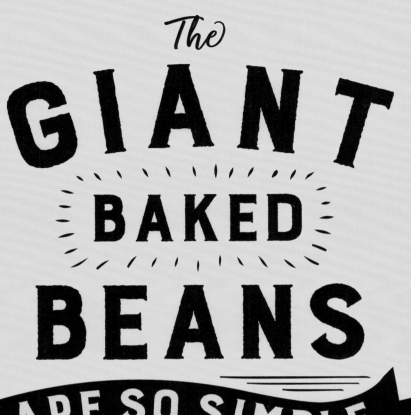

BAKED

BEANS

ARE SO SIMPLE

I ACTUALLY PREFER
THEM *to* BAKED BEANS!

KATRINA

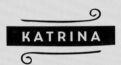

Everyone in my house
loves **HASH BROWN
BREAKFAST BAKE**

KEZ

**EGG-IN-THE-HOLE
BREAKFAST BAGEL is**
so *tasty* and filling.

EMMA

GLAMORGAN SAUSAGES

🕐 **10 MINS** | 🍳 **33 MINS** | ✗ **SERVES 8**

Glamorgan sausage is a Welsh vegetarian recipe made up of cheese, leeks, breadcrumbs and herbs. Our version uses low-fat Cheddar and cooking spray to keep the calories down. The sausages can be served as a snack with a dipping sauce, or as part of a full veggie breakfast. Either way, they taste incredible!

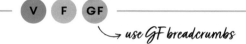

↳ use GF breadcrumbs

PER SERVING:
158 KCAL
13G CARBS

low-calorie cooking spray
2 leeks, green and white parts
    washed and very finely chopped
120g wholemeal breadcrumbs
160g reduced-fat Cheddar,
    finely grated
3 tsp mustard powder
1 tsp garlic granules
1 tsp dried thyme
½–1 tsp xanthan gum
2 eggs, one for the mix and
    one beaten for basting
sea salt and freshly ground
    black pepper

TO ACCOMPANY *(optional)*
Ketchup Tomatoes, page 221 and
    Cauliflower Tots, page 229
    (+ 202 kcal per serving)

Preheat the oven to 220°C (fan 200°C/gas mark 7).

Place a frying pan over a medium heat, spray with low-calorie cooking spray and add the leeks. Gently cook for 3 minutes, until the leeks have softened.

Add the cooked leeks to a bowl and mix in the breadcrumbs, cheese, mustard powder, garlic, thyme, ½ teaspoon xanthan gum and one of the eggs. You should have a thick, heavy dough. Add another ½ teaspoon xanthan gum if it is still a bit crumbly. Split into eight equal-sized balls and roll into long sausage shapes – make sure they are all the same thickness so that they will cook at the same rate.

Spray a foil-lined baking tray with low-calorie cooking spray. Place the sausages on the tray and baste the tops with half of the remaining egg. Spray the tops of the sausages with low-calorie cooking spray and place them in the middle of the oven for 15 minutes.

Gently turn the sausages over and baste with the rest of the egg. Spray with more low-calorie cooking spray and cook for a further 15 minutes.

Remove from the oven and serve hot. The sausages can be frozen once cooled. Defrost fully before reheating in the oven.

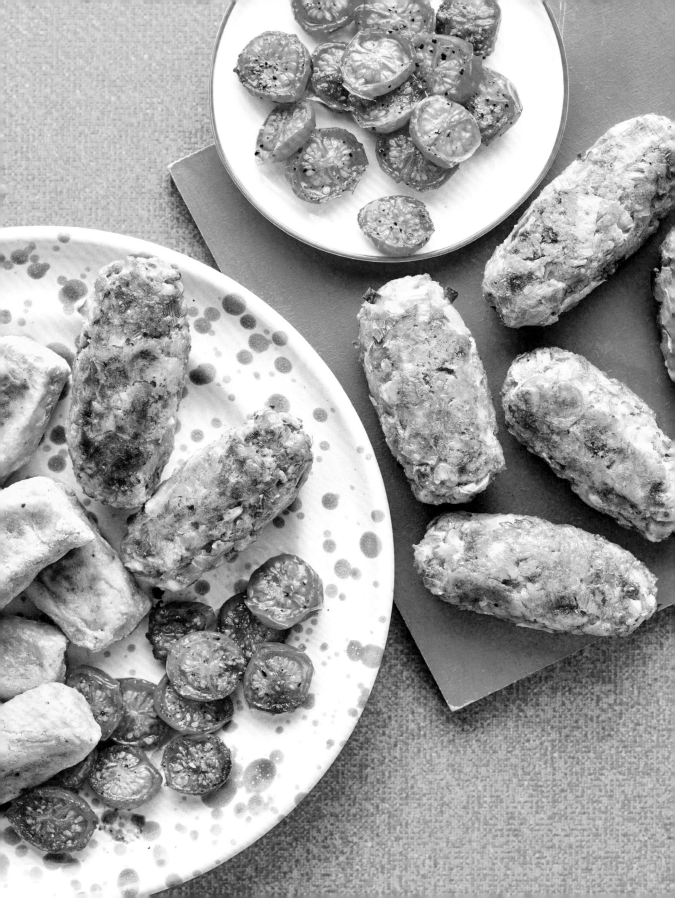

GIANT BAKED BEANS

🕐 **5 MINS** | 🍲 **10 MINS** | ✕ **SERVES 4**

Baked beans are a cupboard staple, but did you know that the average tin contains up to 3 teaspoons of added sugar? We think it's much tastier (and healthier) to make your own with butter beans – plus everything is better when it's oversized! You could also add a little bit of spice or switch the butter beans for haricot for more traditional-style baked beans.

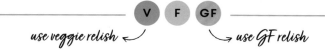

use veggie relish ↜ V F GF ↝ *use GF relish*

PER SERVING:
144 KCAL
24G CARBS

2 x 400g tins butter beans, drained
1 x 500g carton passata
1 tbsp Worcestershire sauce
   or Henderson's relish
1 tsp balsamic vinegar
½ tsp sweet paprika
1 tsp onion granules
½ tsp garlic granules
¼ tsp mustard powder
½ tsp granulated sweetener
sea salt and freshly ground
   black pepper

In a saucepan add the butter beans and passata. Add the Worcestershire sauce, balsamic vinegar, paprika, onion granules, garlic granules, mustard powder, sweetener and some salt and pepper. Give the beans a stir and gently simmer over a low heat with the saucepan lid on for 10 minutes, stirring occasionally.

Serve on toast, with an egg, on the side of a fry-up – the possibilities are endless. The beans can be frozen once allowed to cool.

Tip

Don't confuse onion granules for onion salt – the dish will be far too salty if you use the wrong one. The same applies to garlic granules.

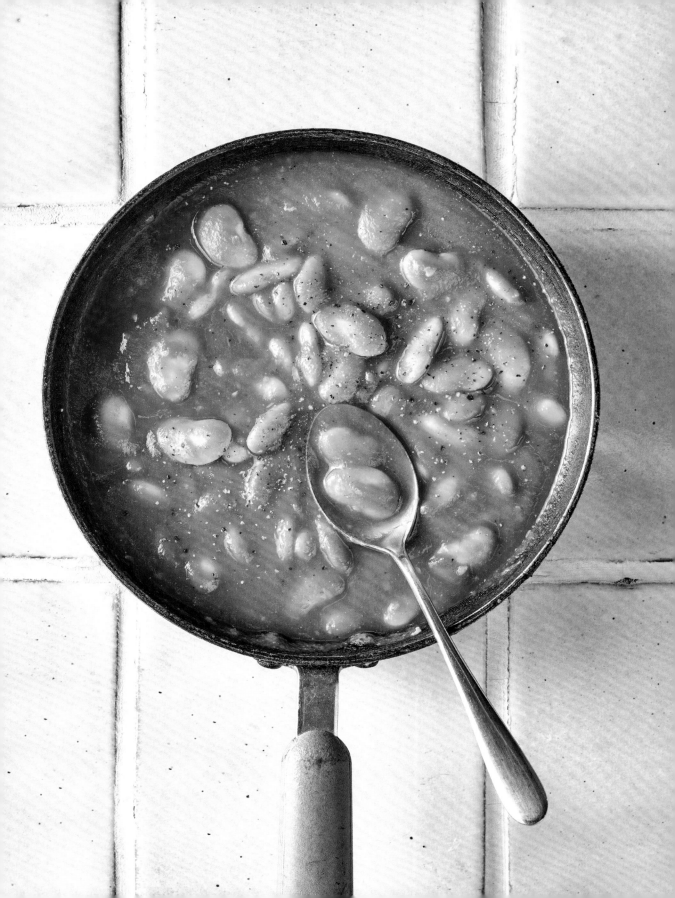

HASH BROWN BREAKFAST BAKE

🕐 **10 MINS** | 🍲 **22 MINS** | ✕ **SERVES 6**

An all-in-one cooked breakfast with a crispy hash brown topping? Yes please! Such a simple dish, but it feels so naughty. Keep your meats lean and the calories will look after themselves. It's basically a full English breakfast without the washing up and for only 189 calories – absolute winner! Swap the tinned baked beans for two portions of our Giant Baked Beans (page 36) if you like; this will make the calorie-count even lower.

F **GF**

→ *use GF relish*

PER SERVING:
189 KCAL
23G CARBS

2 baking potatoes (about
   170g each), diced into
   1–2cm (½–¾ in) cubes
250ml water
low-calorie cooking spray
2 small onions, peeled and diced
8 bacon medallions, chopped into
   small pieces
8 mushrooms, sliced
1 tsp Worcestershire sauce
   or Henderson's relish
sea salt and freshly ground
   black pepper
1 x 400g tin baked beans
1 tsp garlic granules
2 tsp onion granules

Tip

You can prepare this the night before. Keep covered in the fridge and save the final step – cooking in the oven – for the morning.

Preheat the oven to 220°C (fan 200°C/gas mark 7).

Put the potatoes into a microwavable bowl with the water. Microwave on high for 7 minutes.

While the potatoes are cooking, spray a frying pan with low-calorie cooking spray. Add the onions, bacon and mushrooms with the Worcestershire sauce and fry for 5 minutes, until the onions have softened and the bacon is cooked. Season with salt and pepper to taste, remembering that bacon is quite salty.

Once the bacon mix is cooked, spoon it into the bottom of an ovenproof dish. You can do this in one large dish or across six individual ones. Pour the baked beans over the top of the bacon mix.

When the potatoes are ready, they should be cooked through but still hold their shape. Drain the water off, coat with low-calorie cooking spray, sprinkle over the garlic granules and onion granules and season with salt and pepper to taste. Lay the potato cubes over the baked beans, making sure to cover the top in a layer. Spray the potatoes with low-calorie cooking spray.

Place the ovenproof dish(es) in the middle of the hot oven for 15 minutes, until the potatoes on top are golden and crispy. Remove from the oven and serve. The bake can be frozen once allowed to cool (defrost fully before reheating).

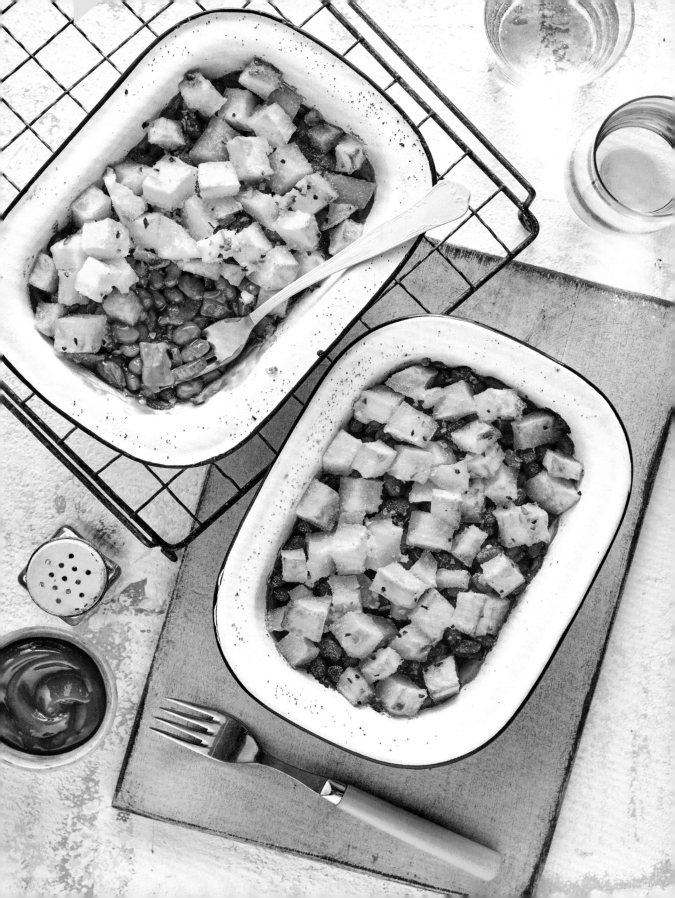

ROSTI WAFFLE *with* ASPARAGUS *and* POACHED EGG

🕐 **15 MINS** | 🗑 **25 MINS** | ✕ **SERVES 2**

Waffles are always such a great breakfast staple. Filling and tasty, this potato waffle can be topped with almost anything you have in the cupboard, but we've gone for some tasty asparagus and a gooey, melty poached egg for a really decadent breakfast that takes around half an hour to put together. Perfect for a lazy Sunday.

PER SERVING:
281 KCAL
38G CARBS

400g potato, peeled
2 spring onions, trimmed and
  finely chopped
½ tsp garlic salt
low-calorie cooking spray
100g asparagus spears, trimmed
2 eggs
sea salt and freshly ground
  black pepper

Coarsely grate the potato and place it in a clean tea towel. Wrap the tea towel around the potato and squeeze to remove as much of the moisture you can. When it's as dry as possible, place it in a bowl. Add the spring onions and garlic salt. Mix well and form the mixture into a ball.

Turn on your waffle maker, spray the plates with some low-calorie cooking spray, place the potato ball in the middle, then close the lid tightly. Cook on a medium heat for 20 minutes or until cooked and golden brown.

While you're waiting for the waffle, cook the asparagus in a pan of boiling salted water for 5 minutes, then drain and keep the asparagus warm.

Poach the eggs in a pan of simmering salted water for 4 minutes (or longer if you prefer a harder yolk). For easy poached eggs, we like to place a piece of cling film in a ramekin. Crack in an egg, then season before twisting the cling film to make a 'package'. Place the wrapped egg in a pan of simmering water for 4–6 minutes, then open the cling film carefully and remove the cooked egg with a spoon.

When the rosti waffle is cooked, remove from the waffle maker, cut into four and arrange two quarters on plates. Place the cooked asparagus and poached egg on top.

The waffle can also be frozen on its own once cooled. Defrost thoroughly and reheat in the oven to serve.

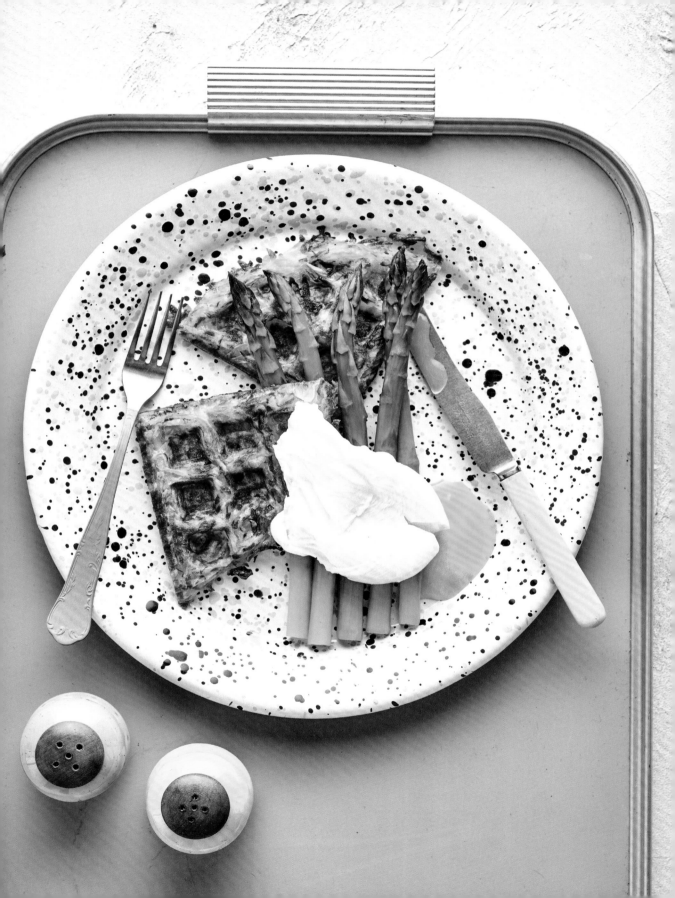

HALLOUMI *and* SMOKY BACON HASH

🕐 **5 MINS** | 🍲 **10 MINS** | ✕ **SERVES 2**

Sunday brunch just got interesting! This savoury dish makes for a filling breakfast, but one that won't leave you feeling guilty for the rest of the day. Ready in only 15 minutes, this hash uses cooking spray instead of drizzles of oil to keep it light. The potatoes and halloumi still crisp up really nicely, and go so well with the sweet flavours of the red pepper and tomatoes.

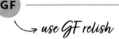

— use GF relish

PER SERVING:
374 KCAL
15G CARBS

90g reduced-fat halloumi
low-calorie cooking spray
4 bacon medallions, diced
100g cooked new potatoes,
    cut in half
100g button mushrooms, halved
½ red pepper, deseeded and cut
    into 1cm (½in) dice
6 cherry tomatoes
1 tsp smoked paprika
¼ tsp garlic granules
1 tsp tomato puree
1 tbsp Worcestershire sauce
    or Henderson's relish
3 tbsp water
30g spinach
2 eggs
sea salt and freshly ground
    black pepper

Cut the halloumi into twelve even-sized pieces. Spray a frying pan with low-calorie cooking spray, add the halloumi and fry over a medium–high heat for 2–3 minutes, until the outside is golden and crisp. Place on a plate and set aside.

Respray the frying pan. Add the bacon, potatoes, mushrooms and pepper, and stir-fry for 3–4 minutes, until the bacon is cooked and the potatoes are starting to brown. Add the cherry tomatoes, smoked paprika and garlic granules, stirring well in order to coat the hash with the spices. Add the tomato puree, Worcestershire sauce or Henderson's relish, and the 3 tablespoons of water. Add the spinach, stir well and turn the heat down to low. Stir in the halloumi.

Spray a second frying pan with low-calorie cooking spray and fry the eggs, until they are cooked to your liking. Taste before seasoning with salt and pepper, as the halloumi and bacon both contain salt.

Divide the hash between two dishes and top each with a fried egg before serving.

MAKE *it* VEGGIE

Leave out the bacon for a veggie hash.

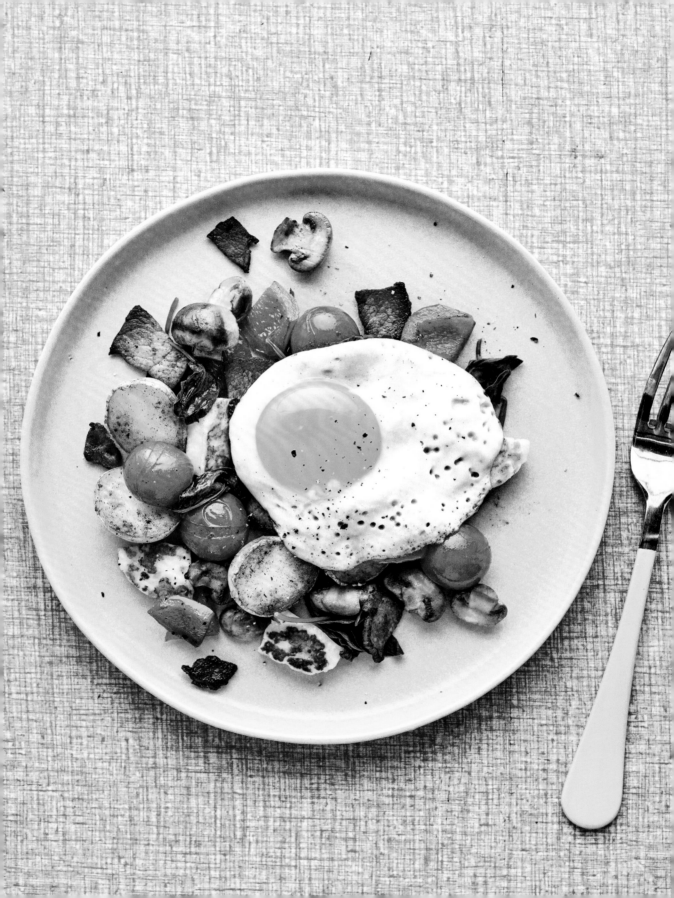

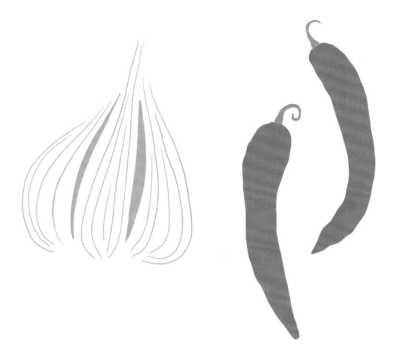

FAKEAWAYS

CRYING TIGER BEEF

🕐 **5 MINS** | 🍲 **4–10 MINS** | ✕ **SERVES 2**

A tasty alternative to a classic steak, this quick Thai recipe combines glazed meat and a saucy salsa to make a delicious dish. Traditionally, this steak would be spicy enough to induce tears, hence the name. However, you can make it as hot as you like by adjusting the amount of chilli in the dressing. Or, you could swap the red chillies for half a red bell pepper if you like. The dressing is very similar to a chimichurri sauce in texture, made with fresh herbs.

GF

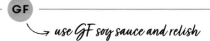 *use GF soy sauce and relish*

PER SERVING:
362 KCAL
12G CARBS

2 extra-lean medallion steaks
  (about 170g each)
2 tbsp reduced-salt soy sauce
1 tbsp Worcestershire sauce
  or Henderson's relish
freshly ground black pepper,
  to taste
low-calorie cooking spray

FOR THE DRESSING
20g fresh coriander, stalks and
  leaves finely chopped
2 tomatoes, finely diced
1–2 red chillies, deseeded and
  finely chopped, or 1–2 tsp
  dried chilli flakes
1 spring onion, trimmed and
  finely chopped
2 garlic cloves, peeled and minced
2 tbsp fish sauce
2 tbsp lime juice or lemon juice
2 tsp granulated sweetener

Place the steaks in a bowl. Pour over the soy sauce and Worcestershire sauce, season with some black pepper and leave to marinate for a few minutes while you make your dressing.

Mix together all the dressing ingredients in a bowl.

Place a frying pan over a medium heat and spray with low-calorie cooking spray. Place the steaks in the pan and pour the marinade left in the bowl on top. Cook the steaks to your preference. The exact times will vary depending on the thickness of your steaks, but it will be around 2 minutes each side for rare, 3 minutes each side for medium and 4 minutes each side for well done. You can check how well done the meat is by pressing the steak with your finger. When you press down, a rare steak will be quite spongy with little resistance, a medium steak will only have a little resistance and a well-done steak will be quite firm.

Once cooked, take the meat out of the pan and leave to rest for a few minutes before slicing and serving with the dressing.

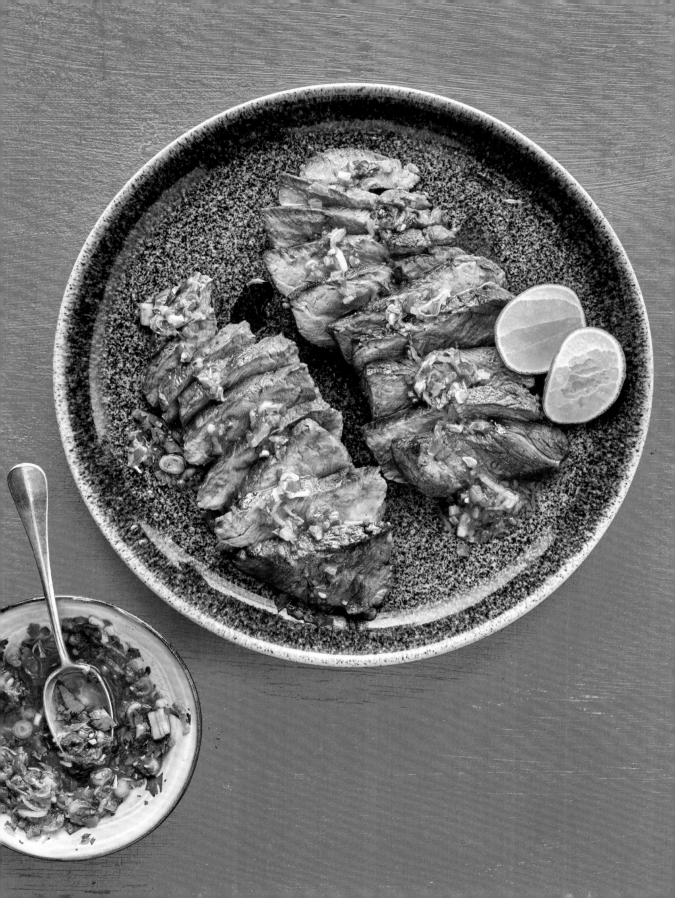

FISH *and* CHIPS

🕐 **15 MINS** | 🍲 **40–50 MINS** | ✕ **SERVES 4**

This is our Pinch of Nom take on the classic British dish, using breadcrumbs to coat the fish instead of a high-calorie batter. This is the ultimate Friday-night fakeaway, and could be enjoyed with a side of our French Peas (see page 226). You could even serve it in newspaper if you want the full fish 'n' chips experience! Friday fish and chips – nothing better!

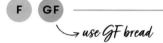

→ *use GF bread*

PER SERVING:
333 KCAL
42G CARBS

800g potatoes, peeled
low-calorie cooking spray
30g wholemeal bread
1 lemon
1 tsp chives, fresh chopped
   or dried
sea salt and freshly ground
   black pepper
4 skinless cod fillets or similar
   (about 150g each)

TO ACCOMPANY *(optional)*
4 x 75g tins mushy peas
   (+ 66 kcal per serving)

Tip

You can freeze the uncooked chips for cooking on a later date.

FOR THE CHIPS

Start with the chips as they take longer to make than the fish.

OVEN METHOD

Preheat the oven to 200°C (fan 180°C/gas mark 6).

Cut the peeled potatoes into 1cm (½in) slices, and then into 1cm (½in) strips to make chips.

Place the potatoes into a large bowl of cold water and rinse well. Drain the water, pat dry with some kitchen towel and spray with low-calorie cooking spray until they are all coated. Season with some salt.

Place onto a non-stick baking tray and cook in the oven for 20 minutes. After 20 minutes, turn the chips over on the baking tray, spray with some more low-calorie cooking spray and return to the oven for a further 15–20 minutes until golden.

AIR FRYER METHOD

Cut the peeled potatoes into 1cm (½in) slices, and then into 1cm (½in) strips to make chips. Place the potatoes in a large bowl of cold water and rinse well.

Continued...

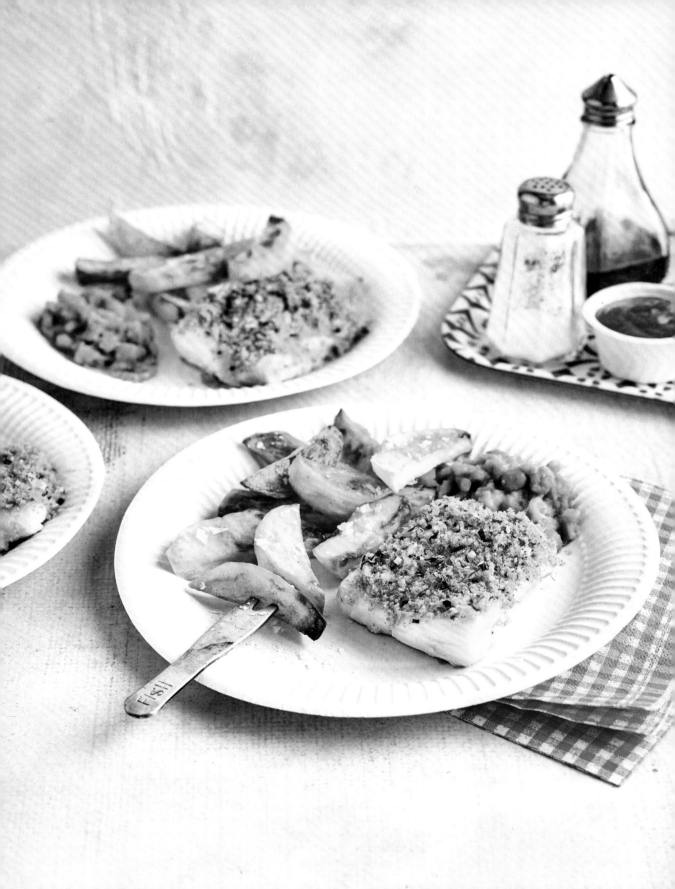

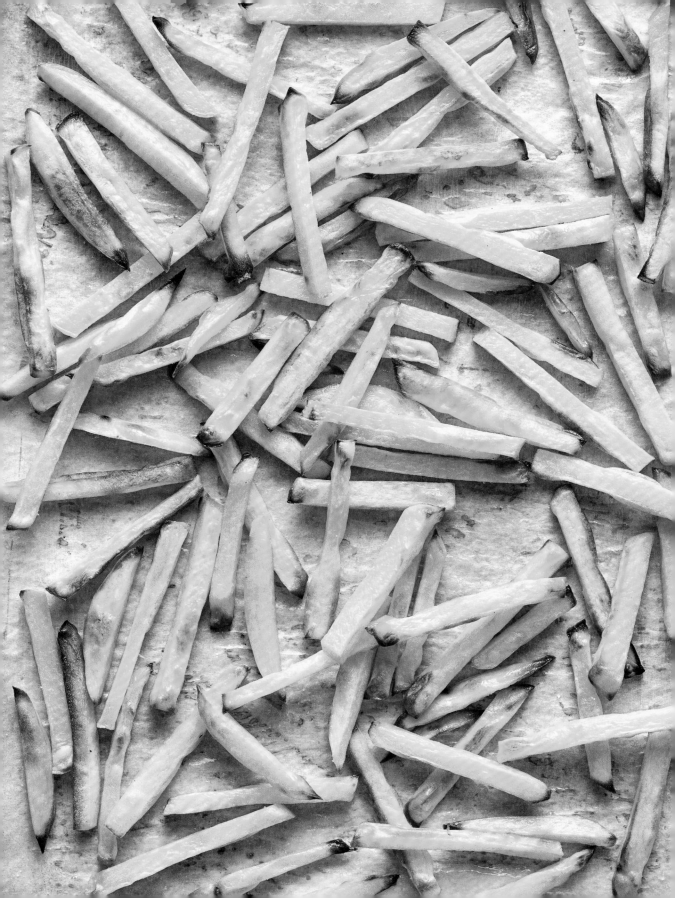

Drain the water, pat dry with some kitchen towel and spray with low-calorie cooking spray until they are all coated. Season with salt.

Place into the air fryer. Set the air fryer to 180°C and cook for 15–20 minutes, shake them around halfway through to make sure they cook evenly. After 15–20 minutes, check to see if the chips are done. If not, cook for a further 5 minutes at a time until they are cooked and golden brown.

FOR THE FISH

Preheat the oven to 200°C (fan 180°C/gas mark 6).

Using a food processor, blitz the bread into fine breadcrumbs and set aside in a bowl. Using a fine grater or zester, remove the zest from the lemon and add it to the breadcrumbs, along with the chives and some salt and pepper. Stir well.

Pat the fish dry using some kitchen towel, then place the fillets on a baking tray that has been sprayed with some low-calorie cooking spray. Season the fish with a little salt and pepper, then divide the breadcrumb topping into four equal portions and place on top of the fish. Pat it down gently to form a crust, and so that it doesn't fall off!

Cook in the oven for about 10 minutes, until the fish is opaque, and serve with the chips.

Tip

You can cut the chips as thinly or thickly as you want (see photo opposite and on page 49). Thinner chips don't need as long in the oven/air fryer so keep an eye on them.

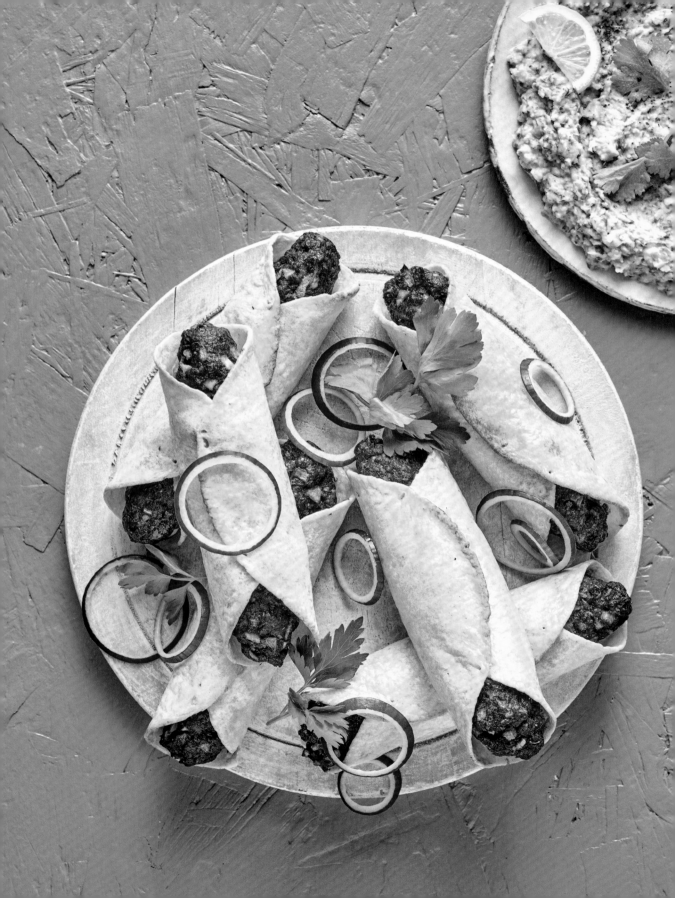

SEEKH KEBAB ROLLS

🕐 **10 MINS** | 🍲 **30 MINS** | ✕ **SERVES 6**

Inspired by a popular Indian street food, this recipe is a cross between a sausage roll and a kebab. We've used low-calorie tortilla wraps to replace the paratha roll, so it's much simpler to make and lower in calories. It's the perfect dish for a fakeaway or a midweek family sharing-meal.

F

PER SERVING:
293 KCAL
25G CARBS

500g 5%-fat minced beef
1 large onion, peeled and
    finely diced
2 tsp garlic granules
1 tsp ground ginger
2 tsp ground coriander
1 tsp dried mint
1 tsp ground cumin
½ tsp chilli powder (hot or
    mild, it's up to you!)
sea salt and freshly ground
    black pepper
low-calorie cooking spray
6 low-calorie tortilla wraps
1 egg, beaten

TO ACCOMPANY *(optional)*
Lemon and Coriander Hummus,
    page 236 (+ 54 kcal per serving)

Tip
This Seekh Kebab recipe also works well without the tortilla, if you want to make them even lighter.

Preheat the oven to 220°C (fan 200°C/gas mark 7).

Add the mince, onion, garlic, ginger, coriander, mint, cumin and chilli powder to a bowl. Season with salt and pepper. Knead the mxiture with clean hands until combined.

Line a baking tray with foil and spray with low-calorie cooking spray. Split the mix into six and shape long sausages out of it. They should be a little longer than the tortilla wraps you are using. Place the kebabs onto the foil, spray the tops with low-calorie cooking spray and place in the oven for 15 minutes. When ready, liquid will have come out onto the tray and the outsides will be browned.

Take a tortilla wrap, baste it with egg and lay a kebab in the middle. Fold the tortilla over, leaving the ends open. If the wrap is too big you can trim it down. Press down gently on the join to seal it. Place the wrapped kebab onto a fresh piece of foil sprayed with low-calorie cooking spray. Repeat with the rest of the kebabs. Baste the tops of the kebabs with more egg, then place back in the oven for 10 minutes until the wrap looks glossy and golden around the edges. Spray the tops with low-calorie cooking spray once more and turn them over. Baste the bottoms with the remaining egg and put back in the oven for a further 5 minutes.

Remove from the oven and serve. These are great cold, making them ideal for lunchboxes, parties and picnics. These can also be frozen once cooled (or frozen raw, once shaped). Defrost thoroughly before cooking or reheating.

CHICKEN TIKKA DRUMSTICKS

🕐 **10 MINS** | 🍲 **40 MINS** | ✗ **SERVES 8**

Chicken Tikka is a popular Indian dish involving marinating the chicken in a spice blend and yoghurt. Just using fat-free yoghurt and cooking the chicken without the usual oils, you'd never guess that these drumsticks, rich in flavour with delicious, juicy chicken, are a healthier version of the usual chicken tikka from the takeaway. For 82 calories per drumstick, they're ideal as a snack or side.

F **GF**

PER DRUMSTICK (WITH DIP):
121 KCAL
7.3G CARBS

8 chicken drumsticks
150g fat-free natural yoghurt, plus extra for serving (optional)
1 tsp smoked paprika
½ tsp ground coriander
½ tsp ground cumin
½ tsp garlic granules
½ tsp garam masala
¼ tsp ground ginger
1 drop of red food colouring (optional)
sea salt and freshly ground black pepper
½ tsp chilli powder (optional)
fresh coriander, to serve (optional)

Preheat the oven to 220°C (fan 200°C/gas mark 7).

Remove the skin from the chicken drumsticks and discard. The easiest way to do this is to pull the skin down to the thin end of the drumstick and then trim off with scissors. Place the drumsticks in a roasting dish.

In a separate bowl mix the yoghurt, paprika, coriander, cumin, garlic granules, garam masala, ginger, food colouring (if using) together and season with salt and pepper. Stir until combined. Pour the yoghurt mix over the drumsticks and make sure you turn them so that they are coated on both sides. Sprinkle the chilli powder over the top of the drumsticks (if using). Put the drumsticks into the middle of the oven for 40 minutes.

Remove from the oven and serve sprinkled with fresh coriander (if using). The drumsticks can also be frozen once cooled. Make sure they are properly defrosted before reheating in the oven.

Tip
If you don't have all the spices, just use 2 tbsp of curry powder instead.

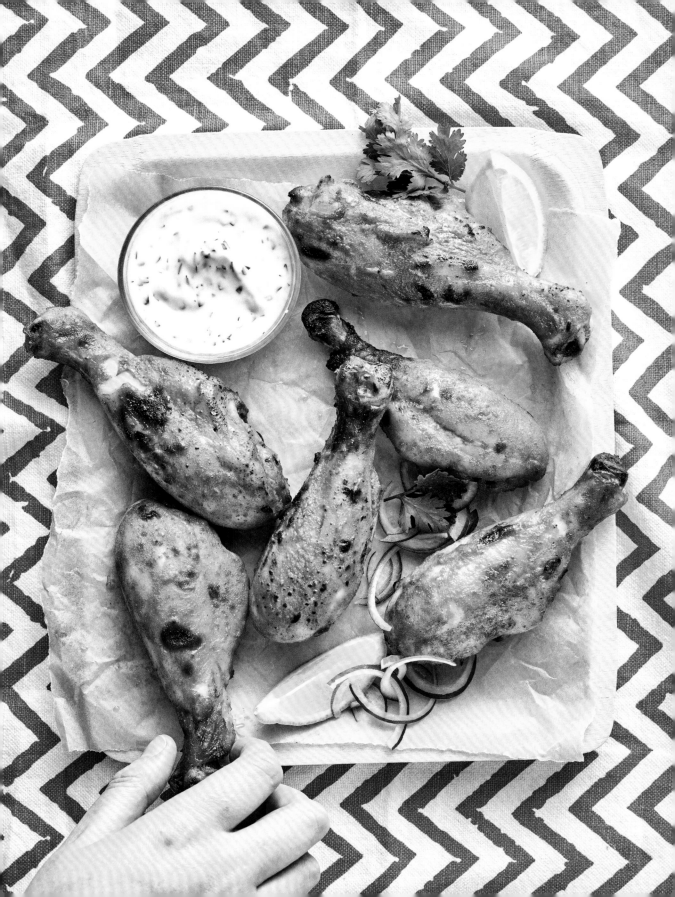

POPCORN CHICKEN

🕐 **5 MINS** | 🍲 **25 MINS** | ✕ **SERVES 2**

There's no need to head to the takeaway for your favourite chicken bites!
Our popcorn chicken is packed full of flavour and you can adjust the spicy
heat to your taste. Serve with a side salad for a complete, tasty meal.

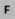

PER SERVING:
356 KCAL
24G CARBS

120g wholemeal bread
½ tsp garlic granules
¼ tsp chilli powder (hot or mild,
    depending on taste)
½ tsp sea salt
300g chicken breast (all skin
    and visible fat removed)
1 egg
low-calorie cooking spray

TO ACCOMPANY *(optional)*
Pink Apple Slaw, page 242
    (+ 40 kcal per serving)

Preheat the oven to 170°C (fan 150°C/gas mark 3). Line a
baking tray with greaseproof paper.

In a mini electric chopper or food processor, blitz the
wholemeal bread into fine crumbs. Place into a shallow dish
with the garlic granules, chilli powder and salt and mix well.

Dice the chicken into bite-sized pieces (about 2cm/¾ in cubes).
Beat the egg in a bowl and add the diced chicken, stirring
to ensure the chicken is coated in egg. Put the chicken into
the breadcrumbs, a few pieces at a time. Shake the chicken
around in the breadcrumbs to coat and place each piece
onto the baking tray. Repeat until all the chicken is coated in
breadcrumbs. If you have any breadcrumbs left over, dip the
breaded chicken into the egg again, then back into the crumbs
for an extra crispy coating!

Spray the chicken with low-calorie cooking spray and pop
in the oven for 20–25 minutes until golden and the chicken pieces
are cooked through. The chicken can also be frozen once cooled
(or frozen raw and coated) – defrost fully before reheating.

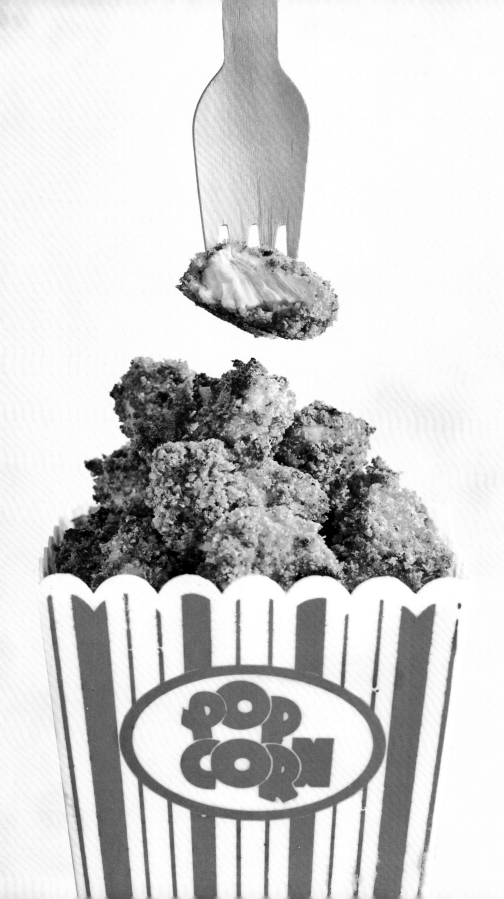

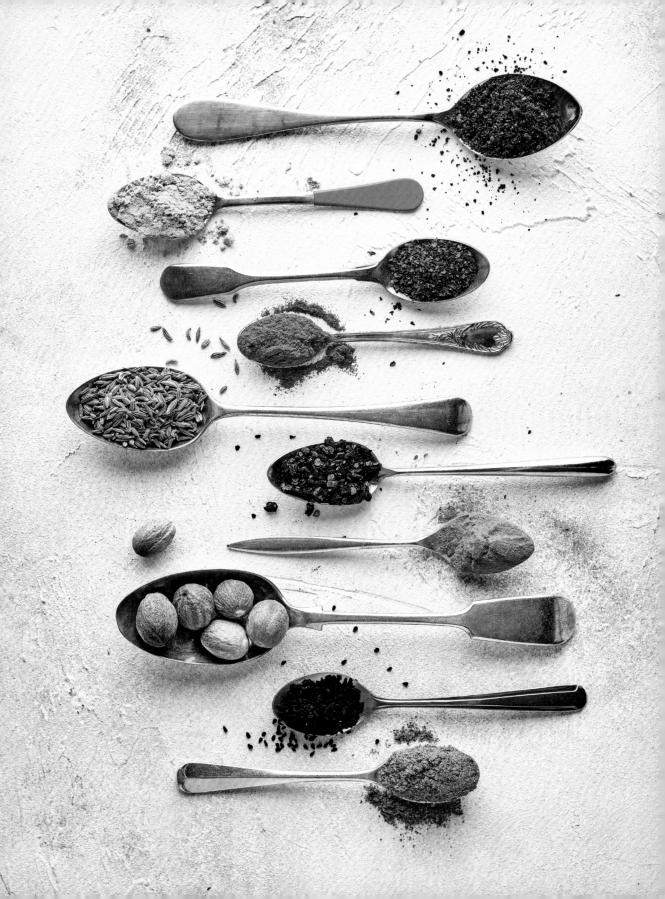

CHICKEN
in
ORANGE
was a
WINNER
IN MY HOUSEHOLD!

CAROLINE

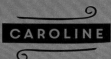

YEUNG CHOW FRIED RICE was bloomin' *lovely!*

FIONA

POPCORN CHICKEN is so *crispy* and *succulent*

JUDITH

CHIPOTLE PORK BURGER

🕐 **5 MINS** | 🍲 **8–10 MINS** | ✕ **SERVES 4**

The lowly burger gets a spicy makeover in this hard-to-believe-the-calories chipotle burger. Making your own burger patty with lean mince is such an easy way to cut out a huge amount of calories in a burger. Swapping to a wholemeal bun, or to gluten-free rolls, means you can up your fibre, but cut out sugar . . . and adding some chipotle spice to your burger? Yassss queen.

F GF

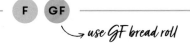
→ *use GF bread roll*

PER SERVING:
355 KCAL
27G CARBS

low-calorie cooking spray
4 x 60g gluten-free seeded
   wholemeal roll
1 red chilli, deseeded and
   thinly sliced, to garnish (optional)

FOR THE BURGERS
500g extra-lean minced pork
4 spring onions, trimmed and
   thinly sliced, plus a little
   reserved for garnish
1 tsp garlic granules
1 tsp chipotle chilli flakes
1 tsp smoked paprika
zest of 1 lime
1 tbsp chopped fresh coriander
sea salt and freshly ground
   black pepper

TO ACCOMPANY *(optional)*
75g mixed side salad
   (+ 15 kcal per serving)
15g 'Lighter than Light' mayonnaise
   (+ 15 kcal per serving)

Place all the burger ingredients in a bowl, season with salt and pepper and mix together until well combined. Divide into four equal-sized portions and shape into burgers, around 1.5cm (½ in) thick. (At this point, you can freeze the burgers to cook on another day – defrost fully before cooking.)

Spray a heavy-based griddle pan with low-calorie cooking spray and place on a high heat. When hot, add the burgers to the pan and cook for 4–5 minutes on each side.

Cut the wholemeal or gluten-free bread rolls in half and if you like, char the cut sides of the rolls on a griddle pan.

Place the burgers in the buns along with some salad and mayonnnaise, and top with spring onion and chilli, if liked.

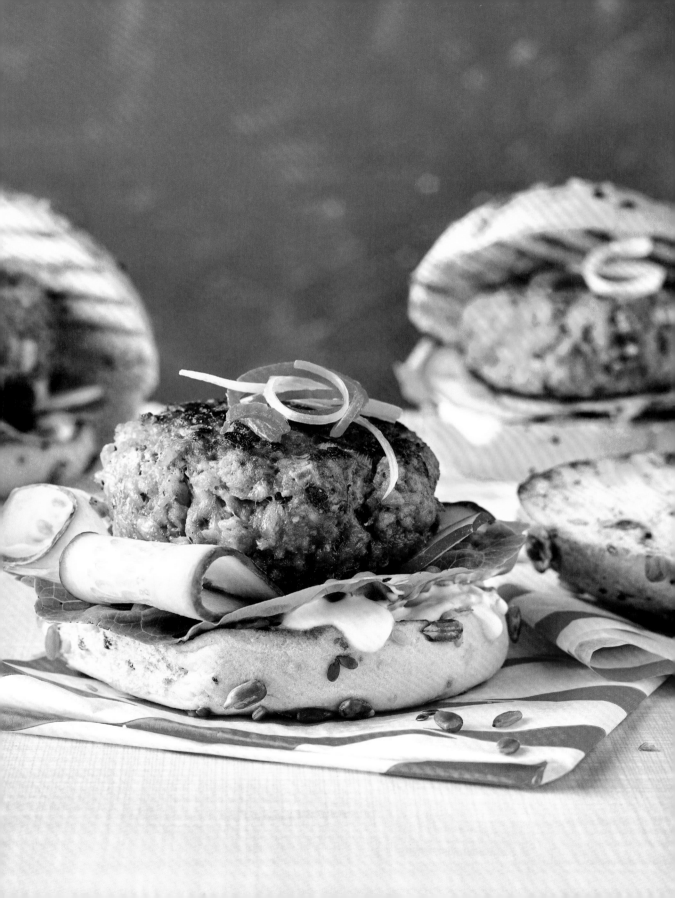

YEUNG CHOW FRIED RICE

🕐 20 MINS | 🍲 20 MINS | ✕ SERVES 4

We love a Chinese takeaway, but we don't love how unhealthy they can be. This Yeung Chow Fried Rice tastes as good as the real thing but comes in at 400 calories per serving. Kerching!

GF → *use GF soy sauce and oyster sauce*

PER SERVING:
400 KCAL
52G CARBS

150g pork loin steaks, cut into strips
200g long-grain rice
1 medium egg, beaten
low-calorie cooking spray
100g frozen peas
bunch of spring onions, trimmed and thinly sliced
1 carrot, peeled and coarsely grated or cut into thin strips (julienne)
100g cooked ham, diced
100g cooked prawns
1 tbsp soy sauce
chilli sauce, to serve (optional)

FOR THE MARINADE
2 tbsp oyster sauce
1 tbsp soy sauce
pinch of Chinese 5-spice
¼ tsp garlic granules

Tip
Substitute 100g of chicken for the prawns, if you wish.

Mix the marinade ingredients together in a bowl, add the pork loin strips and mix until well coated. Cover and refrigerate for 20 minutes.

Cook the rice according to packet instructions, fluff up with a fork, then allow to cool.

Heat a wok over a medium heat and scramble the egg. Place on a plate and put to one side.

Wipe out the wok, spray with low-calorie cooking spray and place over a high heat. Add the marinated pork strips and stir-fry for 5 minutes, until the pork is cooked. Add the peas, onions, ham, carrot and prawns and stir-fry for another minute.

Add the cooked rice, cooked egg and tablespoon of soy sauce. Continue to stir-fry, until the ingredients are well combined and the rice is thoroughly heated, then serve.

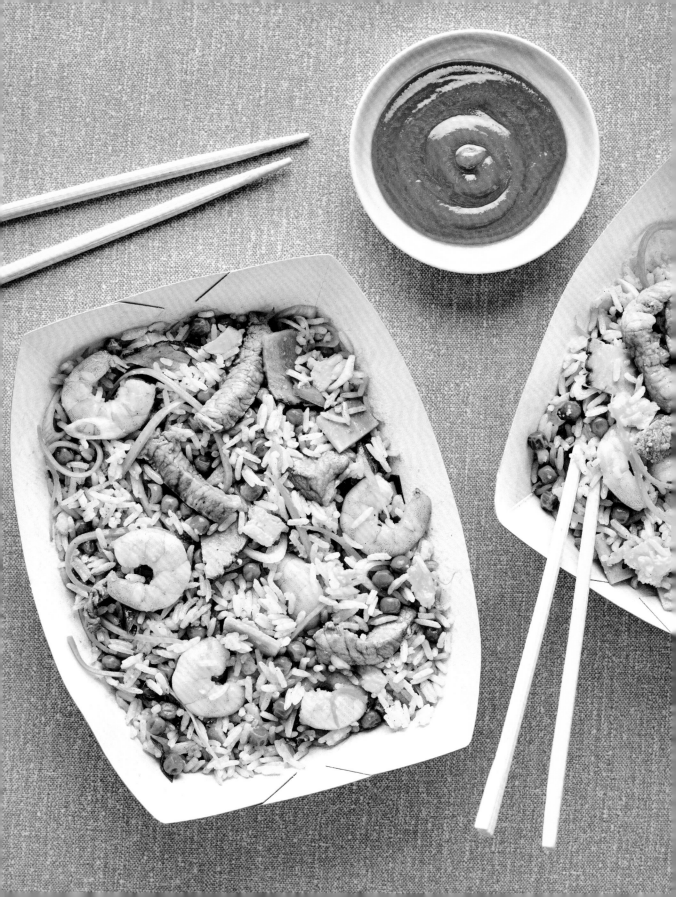

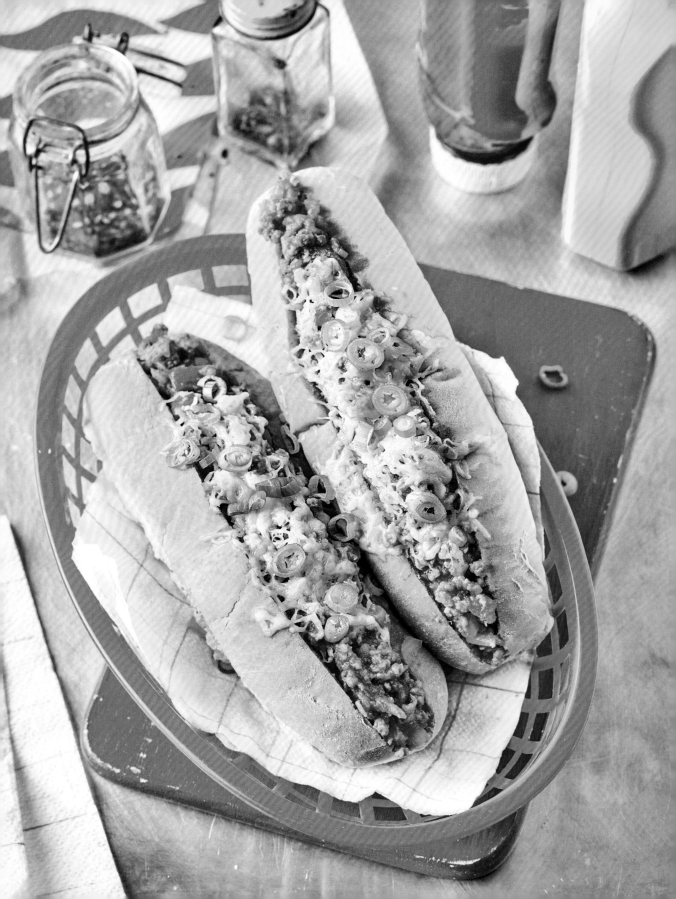

SLOPPY DOGS

🕐 **5 MINS** | 🗑 **20 MINS** | ✕ **SERVES 6**

These Sloppy Dogs are a new take on the hotdog. We've taken lean pork mince and combined it with the flavours of classic toppings, including fried onions, ketchup and mustard. Top it all off with some gooey melted cheese and it's a real dinner winner!

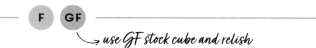

F GF

→ *use GF stock cube and relish*

PER SERVING:
379 KCAL
34G CARBS

2 white onions, peeled and finely chopped
1 red pepper, deseeded and finely chopped
150ml pork stock (2 pork stock cubes dissolved in 150ml boiling water), or use beef or chicken stock
low-calorie cooking spray
500g 5%-fat minced pork
1 tsp onion granules
1 tsp garlic granules
½ tsp sweet paprika
½ tsp mustard powder
2 tsp Worcestershire sauce or Henderson's relish
1 tbsp balsamic vinegar
1 x 400g tin chopped tomatoes
4 tbsp tomato puree
sea salt and freshly ground black pepper
6 gluten-free finger rolls (we like Promise Supersoft White Sandwich Rolls)
120g reduced-fat Cheddar, finely grated
2 spring onions, trimmed and thinly sliced (optional)

Preheat the oven to 220°C (fan 200°C/gas mark 7).

Put the onions, red pepper and the pork stock in a frying pan and sauté over a medium heat. After around 5 minutes the onions will be translucent and the liquid will have reduced to a glossy coating. Spray some low-calorie cooking spray into the pan.

Add the pork mince, onion granules, garlic granules, paprika, mustard powder, Worcestershire sauce and balsamic vinegar. Sauté for 4–5 minutes until the mince has browned.

Once the mince has browned, add the chopped tomatoes and tomato puree. Stir and simmer over a medium–low heat so that it is gently bubbling. After around 5 minutes the sauce should look rich and be reduced and thick. Remember, this is served in a bun, so if the sauce is still runny, reduce it further. Season with salt and pepper to taste. (At this point, if you want to keep the mince for another day, you can freeze it once cooled – defrost fully before reheating.)

Slice the buns down the middle and line up on a baking tray. Spoon the pork mix into the buns and top with the grated cheese. Pop the buns into the oven for 3–5 minutes. You want the cheese to melt but you don't want the buns to burn!

Serve with an optional scattering of spring onions.

CHICKEN *in* ORANGE

🕐 **10 MINS** | 🍲 **10 MINS** | ✗ **SERVES 4**

This dish combines the classic Chinese flavours of a takeaway but ingeniously uses no-added-sugar squash to give it an orange flavour. You'll be pleased to know that you're not pouring a glass of diluted squash into your dish! It simply uses the concentrate to inject that orangey goodness without you needing to reduce an orange sauce for an hour before you can even get cracking on the meal. A super-quick, super-simple fakeaway. Perfect!

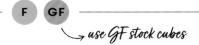

↳ *use GF stock cubes*

PER SERVING:
192 KCAL
7.8G CARBS

low-calorie cooking spray
500g chicken breast (skin and visible fat removed), diced
1 medium onion, peeled and diced
½ red chilli, deseeded and finely diced
500ml chicken stock (2 chicken stock cubes dissolved in 500ml boiling water)
100ml no-added-sugar orange squash
1 tsp onion powder
¾ tsp xanthan gum
1 tsp rice vinegar
1 orange, peeled and cut into segments
4 spring onions, trimmed and thinly sliced

TO ACCOMPANY *(optional)*
50g uncooked rice per portion, cooked according to packet instructions (+ 173 kcal per 125g cooked serving)

Spray a wok with low-calorie cooking spray. Over a high heat, stir-fry the chicken, diced onion and chilli for 4–5 minutes, until the chicken is well browned. Remove to a plate and wipe the pan clean.

Pour the stock, orange squash and onion powder into the wok, return to the heat and bring to the boil. Remove from the heat and add the xanthan gum, ¼ teaspoon at a time, whisking well for a minute between each addition. You may not need the entire amount.

When thickened, add the rice vinegar and return the onions and chicken to the sauce. Return to the heat and simmer for 3–4 minutes, until the chicken is cooked through and no longer pink in the middle.

Stir in the orange segments and spring onions and serve – or you can cool and freeze to keep for another day (defrost fully before reheating).

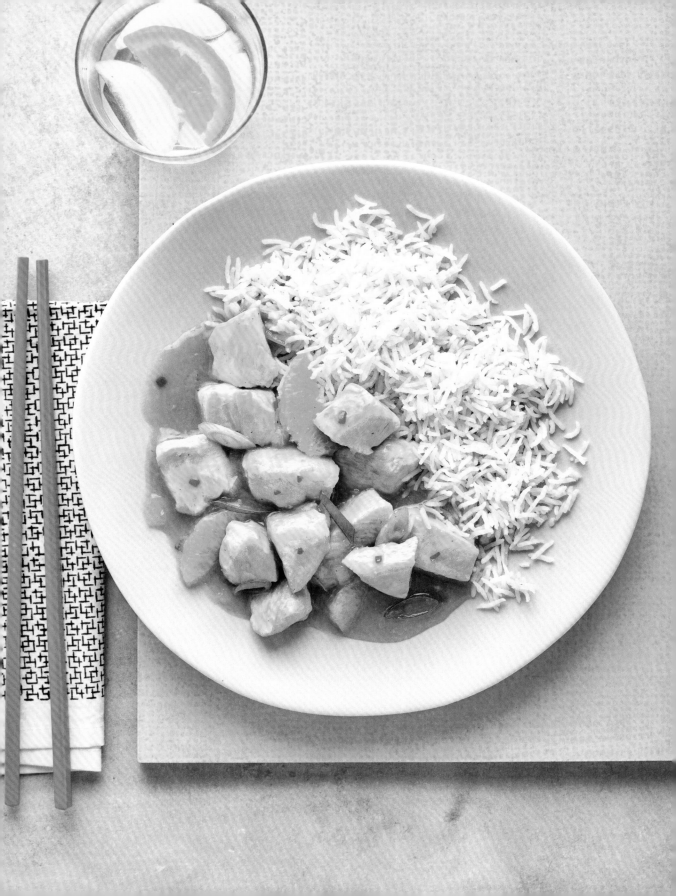

CRISPY TURKEY CHINESE WRAPS

🕐 **5 MINS** | 🍲 **25 MINS** | ✕ **SERVES 4**

Usually made with duck, these crispy wraps are a Chinese staple. Duck, however, can be fatty and expensive. By swapping the duck for a lean meat like turkey, you're getting a very similar taste for fewer calories and less cost – a winning combination, if you ask us.

F

PER SERVING:
255 KCAL
28G CARBS

375g turkey breast steaks
low-calorie cooking spray
4 tsp Chinese 5-spice
4 tbsp dark soy sauce
3 tbsp granulated sweetener
4 tbsp balsamic vinegar
4 low-calorie tortilla wraps
½ cucumber, sliced into batons
6 spring onions, trimmed and
   thinly sliced lengthways

Preheat the oven to 180°C (fan 160°C/gas mark 4).

Place the turkey breast steaks on a baking tray, spray with low-calorie cooking spray and sprinkle over 1 teaspoon of the Chinese 5-spice onto both sides of the steaks. Bake in the oven for 25 minutes, until cooked through and crisp, turning halfway through cooking.

Meanwhile, place the rest of the Chinese 5-spice, dark soy sauce, granulated sweetener and balsamic vinegar in a small saucepan, reserving 2 teaspoons of the balsamic vinegar for the end. Place over a medium heat, stirring regularly, and reduce by half, taking care not to burn the sauce. This will take around 4–5 minutes. Keep warm until ready to serve. If it becomes cool and starts to over-thicken, reheat with a couple of tablespoons of water to loosen.

Once the turkey is cooked, remove it from the oven. (At this point, the turkey can be frozen once cooled – defrost fully before reheating.)

Slice the cooked turkey into strips or shred with forks. Cut the low-calorie tortilla wraps into quarters. Onto each quarter place some crispy turkey, some cucumber and spring onions. Drizzle over a little of the sauce – it is very strong in flavour so a little goes a long way!

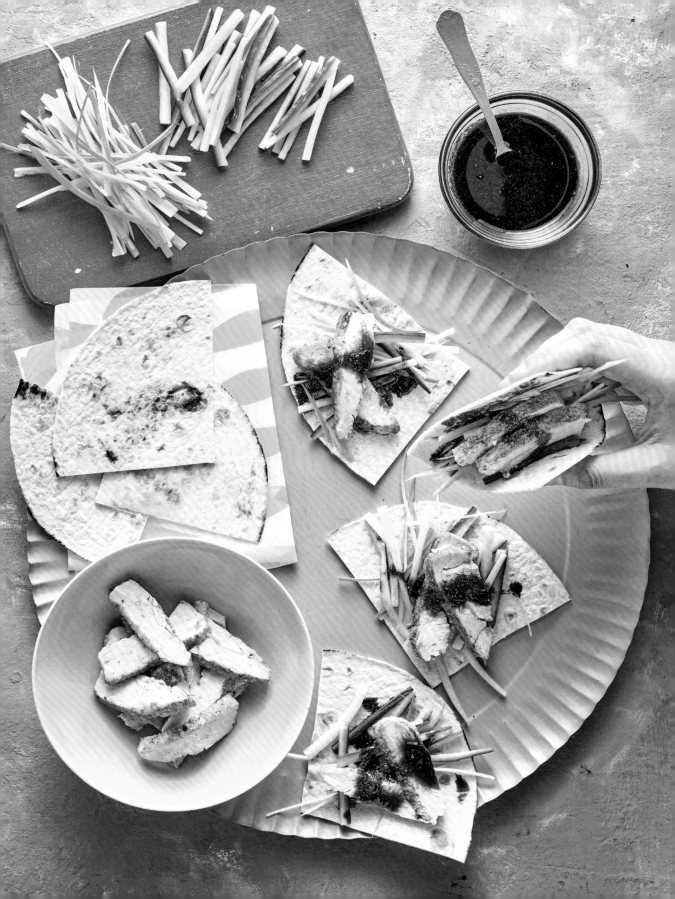

GARLIC *and* LIME BALTI

🕐 **5 MINS** (PLUS MARINATING TIME) | 🍲 **25 MINS** | ✗ **SERVES 4**

As you may be able to tell from the name, garlic and lime take centre-stage in this version of the classic Indian Balti dish. We've kept the spice mild but encourage lovers of heat to crank up the chilli in the curry paste if they wish.

F **GF**

↳ *use a GF stock cube*

PER SERVING:
223 KCAL
18.8G CARBS

500g chicken breasts (skin
   and visible fat removed), diced
4 bell peppers, deseeded and sliced
low-calorie cooking spray
1 x 400g tin chopped tomatoes
150ml chicken stock (1 chicken
   stock cube dissolved in
   150ml boiling water)

FOR THE CURRY PASTE
low-calorie cooking spray
1 small onion, peeled and sliced
6 garlic cloves, peeled and minced
zest and juice of 2 limes, plus extra
   wedges to serve
2 tbsp tomato puree
1 tsp ground turmeric
1 tsp ground coriander
½ tsp ground cumin
½ tsp garam masala
½ tsp ground ginger
¼ tsp chilli powder (or to taste)
½ tsp granulated sweetener
sea salt and freshly ground
   black pepper

TO ACCOMPANY *(optional)*
50g uncooked rice per portion,
   cooked according to packet
   instructions (+ 173 kcal per 125g
   cooked serving)

To make the curry paste, spray the pan with low-calorie cooking spray. Add the onion and garlic and cook over a medium heat for 5 minutes until softened.

Put the cooked onion and garlic in a blender with the rest of the curry paste ingredients and a pinch each of salt and pepper and blend into a paste.

Put the chicken in a bag or bowl with the paste, making sure to coat it well. Marinate the chicken for at least an hour in the fridge.

Once the chicken has been marinated, start on the curry. Add the chicken to a medium frying pan with the peppers and some low-calorie cooking spray. Sauté over a medium heat for 5 minutes, until the peppers have softened and the chicken has browned. Add the tomatoes and stock and simmer over a medium heat for 15 minutes. When it is ready, the chicken will be cooked through and the sauce will have thickened.

Remove the pan from the heat and serve. The curry can also be frozen once cooled – defrost fully before reheating, and make sure it's piping hot all the way through.

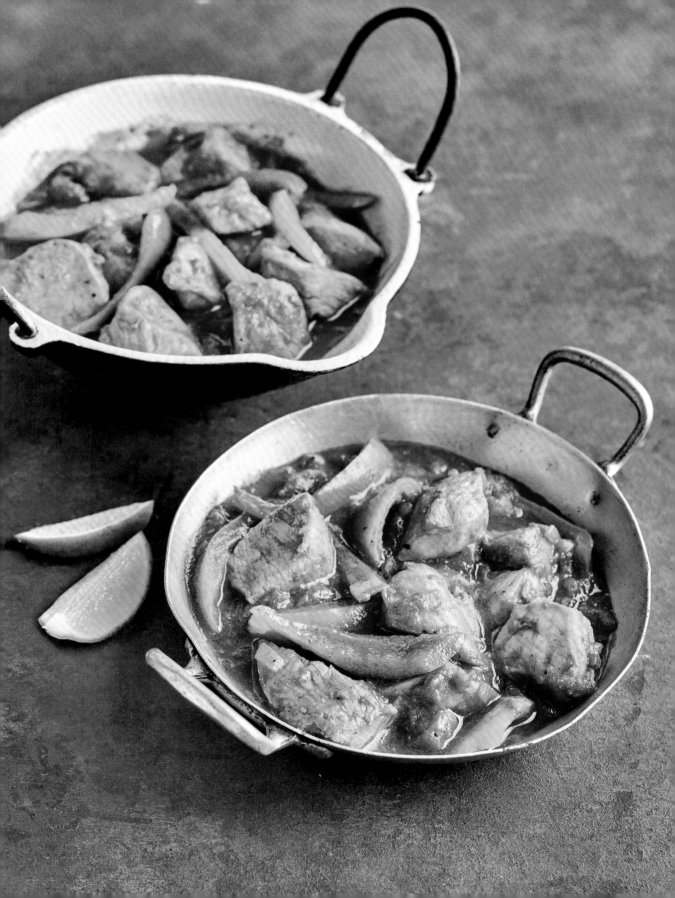

FIRECRACKER PRAWNS

🕐 **10 MINS** | 🍲 **10 MINS** | ✕ **SERVES 4**

This is a great dish to throw together with leftover veg, and tastes just as good as the takeaway version. The combination of oyster and soy sauce gives this recipe an authentic Japanese taste. You can use as little or as much chilli as you like, depending on how much you want to 'firecracker' your prawns!

PER SERVING:
175 KCAL
15G CARBS

low-calorie cooking spray
2 red peppers, deseeded
   and sliced
4 spring onions, finely chopped
1–2 chillies (depending on your
   taste), deseeded and sliced
100g baby corn, cut into 3
100g mangetouts, cut in half
400g raw king prawns, peeled
   and deveined
2 garlic cloves, peeled
   and chopped
4 tbsp oyster sauce
4 tbsp soy sauce
2 tsp tomato puree
juice of ½ lime
½ tsp granulated sweetener
   (or use sugar if you prefer)

TO ACCOMPANY (optional)
1 nest of egg noodles, cooked
   according to packet instructions
   (+ 129 kcal per serving)

Spray a wok with low-calorie cooking spray and stir-fry the peppers, spring onions, chillies, baby corn and mangetouts over a medium–high heat for 2–3 minutes. Add the prawns and continue to cook for another 3–4 minutes, until the prawns turn pink and become opaque.

Add the garlic, oyster sauce, soy sauce, tomato puree, lime juice and sweetener. Stir well and cook for another minute, until you have a thick sauce coating the prawns.

Serve with the egg noodles or your choice of accompaniment.

Tip
Substitute the
prawns for
chicken.

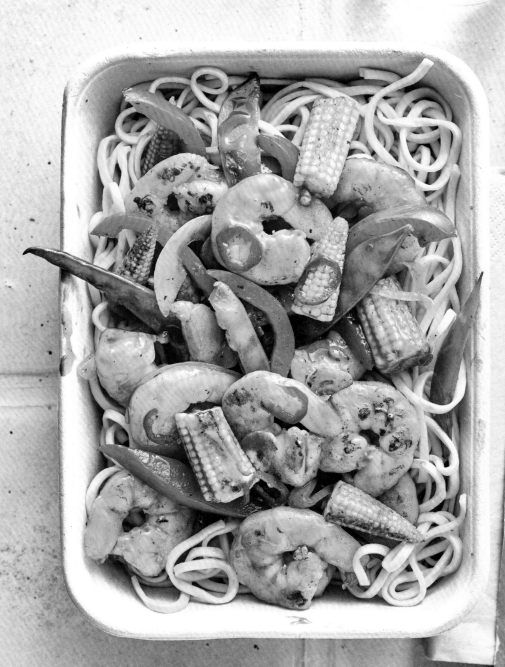

PIZZA-LOADED FRIES

🕐 **5 MINS** | 🍲 **35 MINS** | ✗ **SERVES 2**

There's no need to worry about deciding between pizza or fries with this recipe, as you can have both together! Pizza-loaded Fries combine two favourite takeaways into one, minus the grease and calorific oils. We've used our favourite vegetable pizza topping, but you could use whatever you have in the fridge – top with cheese and nom, nom, nom!

PER SERVING:
390 KCAL
55G CARBS

500g white potatoes
low-calorie cooking spray
1 x 250g carton passata
2 tsp garlic granules
1 tsp onion granules
1 tsp dried oregano
1 tsp dried basil
½ tsp granulated sweetener
sea salt and freshly ground
    black pepper
80g grated mozzarella
¼ small red pepper, deseeded
    and sliced
2 button mushrooms, sliced

Preheat the oven to 180°C (fan 160°C/gas mark 4) and line a baking tray with greaseproof paper.

Peel the potatoes. Cut each potato into slices which are around 5mm (¼ in) thick, and then cut each slice into fries that are also around 5mm (¼ in) thick. Place the fries onto the lined baking tray, spray with low-calorie cooking spray and pop in the oven for 20 minutes until turning golden. (You could also cook your fries in an air fryer for around 16 minutes.)

Meanwhile, into a bowl, add the passata, garlic granules, onion granules, oregano, basil and granulated sweetener, and season with salt and pepper to taste. Mix well.

Once the fries are beginning to turn golden, transfer to the baking dish (or dishes, if making individual portions). Pour over most of the tomato sauce, keeping some aside for dipping, sprinkle over the grated mozzarella and add the slices of pepper and mushrooms – you can add whatever pizza toppings you like.

Put back into the oven for 15 minutes until the cheese has melted and is turning golden. Put the remaining tomato sauce in a small bowl for dipping. The pizza-loaded fries can also be frozen once cooled – defrost fully before reheating.

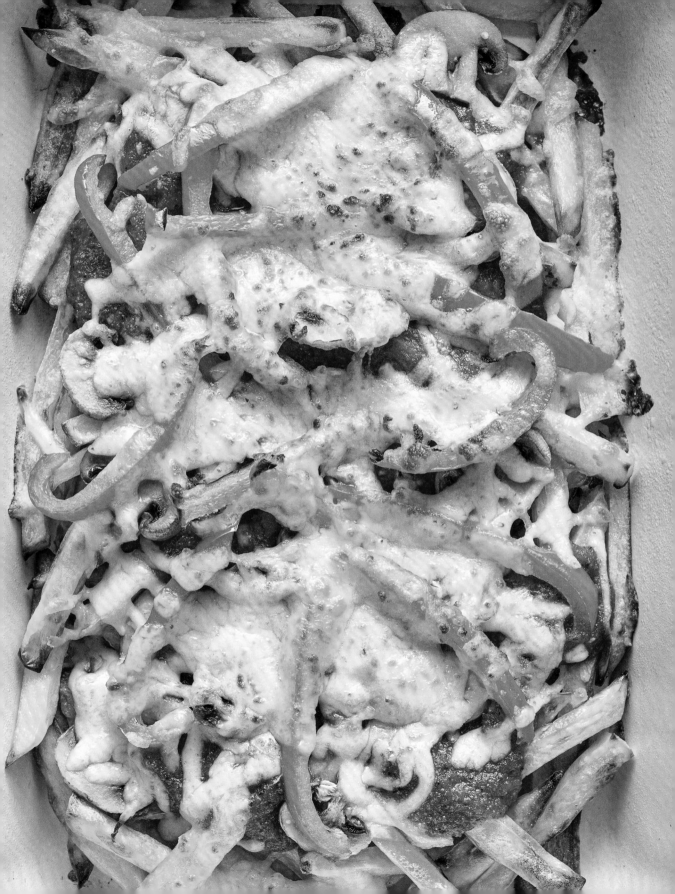

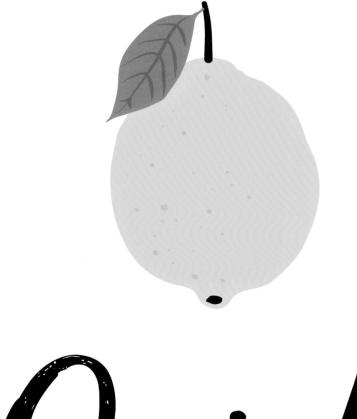

Quick
MEALS

ORANGE, CARROT *and* BEETROOT SALAD

⏱ **15 MINS** | 🍲 **NO COOK** | ✕ **SERVES 2**

This salad not only tastes amazing but it looks incredible on the plate too. The zesty sweetness of the orange paired with the earthy, slightly bitter taste of beetroot doesn't sound like it would match but trust us, you won't look back. Beetroot season in the UK is early July, making this salad a great one to bring to your next summer BBQ!

 V GF

PER SERVING:
63 KCAL
11G CARBS

1 large orange
¼ tsp peeled and grated
    root ginger
1 tsp red wine vinegar
sea salt
60g raw beetroot, peeled and
    cut into thin strips (julienne)
60g carrot, peeled and cut into
    thin strips (julienne)
½ tbsp chopped fresh coriander

Remove the zest from the orange, using a fine grater or zester, and set aside. Then, using a sharp knife, cut off the top and bottom of the orange. Cut the skin away from the flesh in downward strokes. Squeeze any juice from the skin and set aside along with the zest.

Cut between the membranes to segment the orange, reserving any juice. Squeeze any remaining juice out of the leftover membranes.

In a large bowl mix together the ginger, red wine vinegar, 1 teaspoon of the orange zest and 2 tablespoons of the orange juice. Add a little pinch of salt to taste. Stir well, then add the orange segments, beetroot, carrot and coriander.

Stir again and keep refrigerated until you're ready to serve.

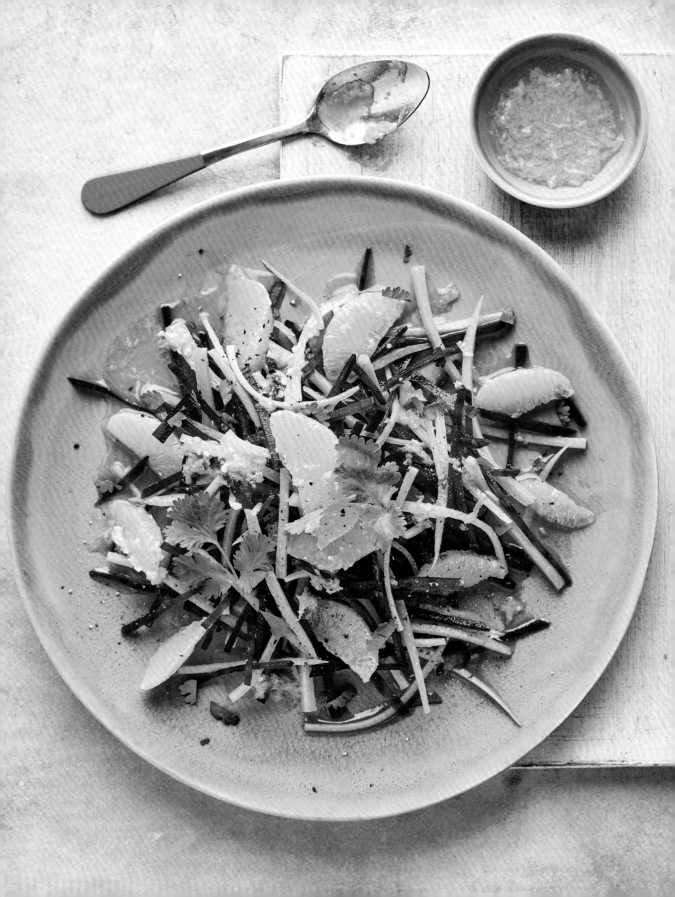

MELT-*in-the*-MIDDLE FISHCAKES

🕐 **20 MINS** | 🍲 **25 MINS** | ✕ **SERVES 4**

Homemade fishcakes are one of the most comforting meals ever, and they are also a really thrifty way of eating fish. Our recipe combines a melting cheese centre with some smoked fish – the perfect duo! These would be great served with some steamed vegetables.

F GF

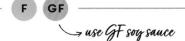
↳ *use GF soy sauce*

PER SERVING:
273 KCAL
24G CARBS

500g potatoes, peeled and
  chopped
250g smoked white fish (such
  as smoked haddock or
  smoked basa)
1 medium egg
2 tbsp finely chopped chives
sea salt and freshly ground
  black pepper
110g light spreadable or
  squeezy cheese
4 Babybel cheeses, wax
  outer coating removed
  and cheese grated
low-calorie cooking spray

TO ACCOMPANY *(optional)*
75g mixed side salad
  (+ 15 kcal per serving)

Preheat the oven to 180°C (fan 160°C/gas mark 4) and line a baking tray with greaseproof paper.

Cook the potatoes in boiling salted water for 20 minutes; they will be cooked when a knife slides easily into the centre. Just before the potatoes are ready, bring a large saucepan of water to the boil and place the fish into the boiling water. Reduce the heat and poach gently for 7 minutes. Once cooked, remove from the water and pat dry to remove any excess liquid.

Drain the cooked potatoes well and mash. Add the mashed potatoes to a bowl and mix in the egg. Flake the fish into the bowl of potato and add the chopped chives. Season to taste, remembering that the smoked fish has its own saltiness.

Put the cheese spread and grated Babybel cheese into a small bowl and mix well. Place a large frying pan on a moderate heat and spray with low-calorie cooking spray.

Split the potato mix into four. With damp hands, pick up one quarter and shape it into a ball. Flatten out slightly and press a quarter of the Babybel cheese and cheese spread mix into the centre. Carefully fold the potato mix around the cheese, ensuring that there are no gaps. This is a little fiddly, so just take your time.

Add each fishcake carefully to the frying pan as they're made. Leave to cook over a gentle heat for 5 minutes before carefully turning and cooking for 5 minutes on the other side.

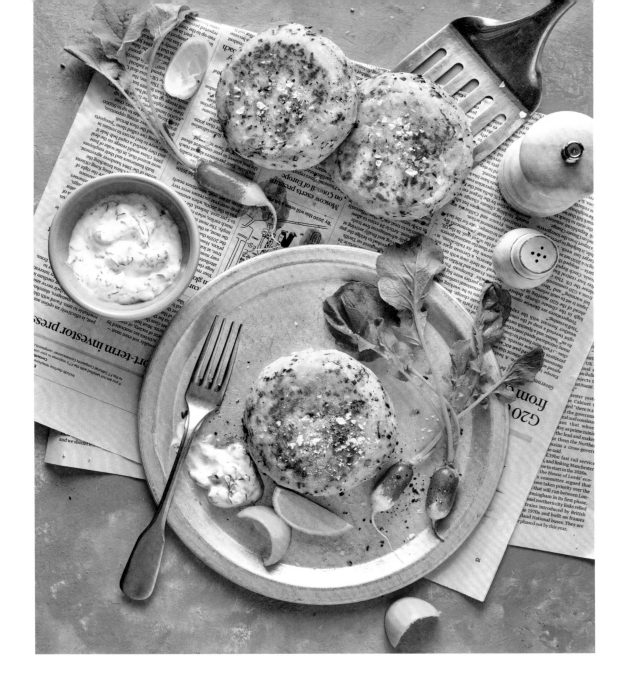

Gently place on the lined baking tray and cook in the oven for 10–15 minutes until the middle is oozing and melted, and the tops are golden. When they are cooked the middle should feel super soft and may appear slightly sunken where the cheese has fully melted.

Serve hot with your choice of accompaniment. The fishcakes can also be frozen once cooled – defrost fully before reheating until piping hot throughout.

CAULIFLOWER-BASE PIZZA

🕐 **10 MINS** | 🍲 **35 MINS** | ✕ **SERVES 2**

We're always on a quest for the perfect guilt-free pizza. We think this comes pretty close! Ingeniously using cauliflower as a base, you'll have no regrets tucking into this veggie-friendly pizza. In fact, you can eat a whole half of it. Half a pizza for 340 calories? Winner.

use a veggie hard cheese

PER SERVING:
340 KCAL
16G CARBS

1 small head of cauliflower, trimmed
60g Parmesan, finely grated
1 large egg
2 tsp xanthan gum
1 x 150g carton passata
1 tsp garlic granules
½ tsp onion granules
½ tsp dried oregano
½ tsp dried basil
½ tsp salt
½ tsp granulated sweetener
80g grated mozzarella
small amounts of sliced pepper, mushrooms and red onion

TO ACCOMPANY *(optional)*
75g mixed side salad
(+ 15 kcal per serving)

Preheat the oven to 180°C (fan 160°C/gas mark 4). Line a large baking tray – a 29cm (11½in) round pizza tray is ideal – with greaseproof paper.

Place the cauliflower into a food processor and blitz until it's the consistency of rice. Put into a microwaveable bowl, cover with cling film and microwave on high for 4 minutes. Allow to cool slightly, then use a clean tea towel or fine sieve to squeeze out any excess moisture. Put the cauliflower in a bowl.

Add the Parmesan, egg and xanthan gum to the cauliflower and mix well. Leave to sit for 2 minutes, then turn out onto the lined baking tray.

Press the cauliflower mix into a circle – the diameter should be 29cm (11½in) – ensuring that the depth of the layer is even. Put in the oven to cook for 15 minutes until just turning golden.

Meanwhile, make the tomato sauce by putting the passata, garlic granules, onion granules, oregano, basil, salt and sweetener in a bowl. Mix well and set aside.

When the pizza base has finished cooking, take it out of the oven. Spread the tomato sauce over the base and sprinkle over the grated mozzarella. Top with your choice of toppings – red pepper, mushrooms and onions work well – and return to the oven for another 10–15 minutes until the cheese is melted and bubbling. Cut into slices and serve.

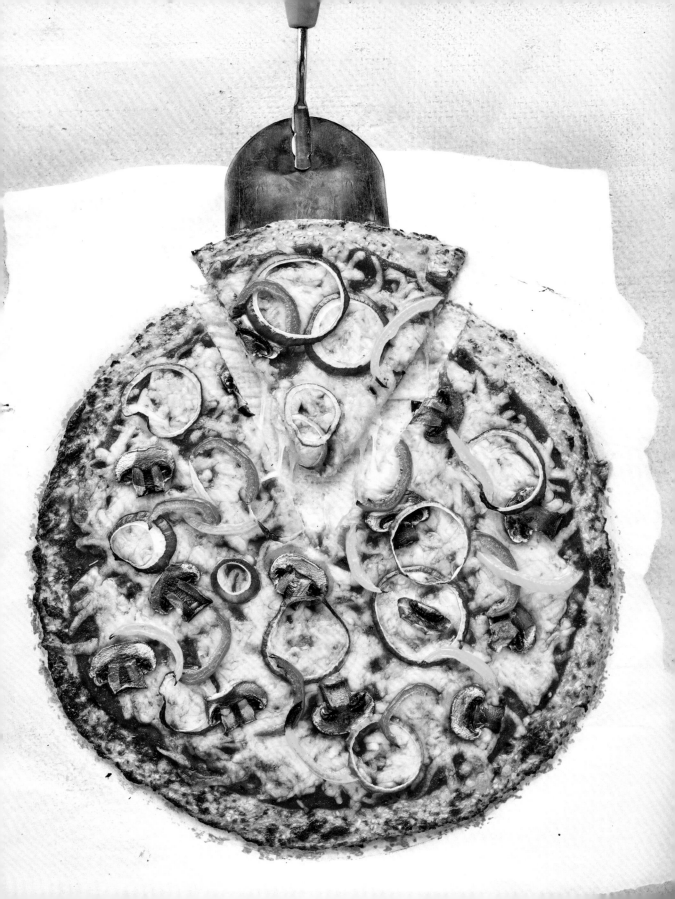

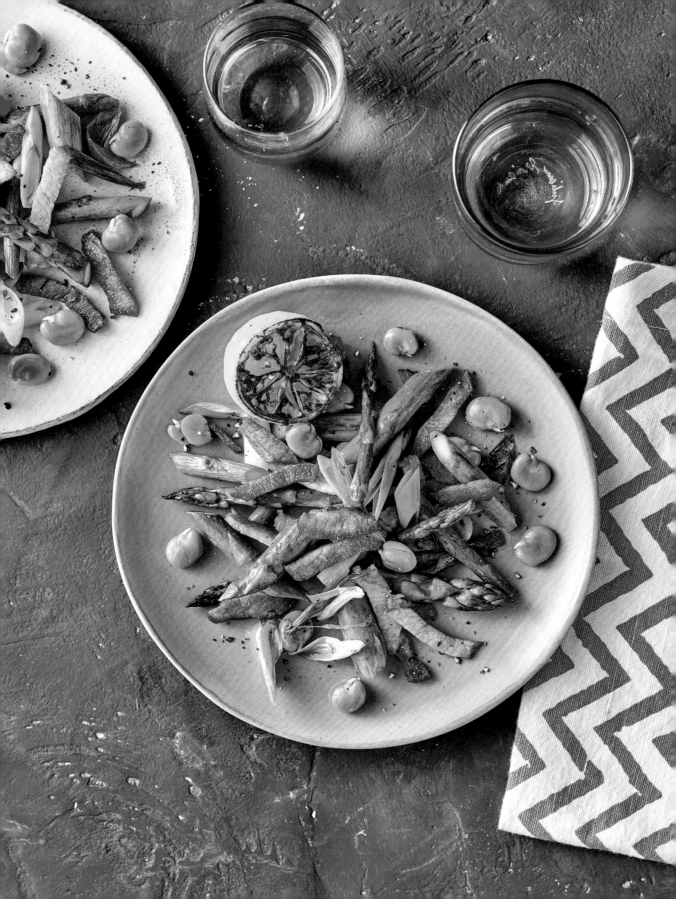

ASPARAGUS, BROAD BEAN
and BACON SALAD

🕐 **5 MINS** | 🍲 **15 MINS** | ✕ **SERVES 2**

A warm salad is one of life's true gifts. This one is given filling power with the broad beans and asparagus. Add some salty bacon, balance it out with the lemony, garlicky dressing and this salad is lifted to tasty heights that can be enjoyed whatever the weather.

GF

PER SERVING:
177 KCAL
8.4G CARBS

75g frozen broad beans
low-calorie cooking spray
4 bacon medallions, cut into strips
2 spring onions, trimmed
   and sliced
1 garlic clove, peeled and chopped
160g asparagus spears, trimmed
   and cut into 3 pieces
juice of ½ lemon
sea salt and freshly ground
   black pepper

Cook the broad beans in boiling water for 5 minutes, drain and place to one side.

Spray a frying pan with low-calorie cooking spray and place over a medium heat. Add the bacon and spring onions, and cook for 2–3 minutes. Next, add the garlic and the asparagus. Continue to sauté for another 4–5 minutes then add the broad beans and squeeze in the lemon juice.

Continue to cook for a further 2 minutes, until the beans are reheated and the asparagus is cooked, but still crunchy.

Taste and season with salt and pepper as required.

Tip

Charring lemons helps to release their juices. Lightly spray the half lemon with low-calorie cooking spray and place it, cut side down, on a hot grill or frying pan for about 3–4 minutes.

BROCCOLI, CHILLI *and* KING PRAWN STIR FRY

🕐 **5 MINS** | 🍲 **12 MINS** | ✕ **SERVES 4**

A stir fry is such a simple and quick, flavourful dish that it almost feels like cheating. Adding the broccoli into the mix makes it very filling, so you might feel you don't need to add noodles or rice. However, at only 143 calories per portion, you can easily add an accompaniment without stretching on the calories.

GF

↳ *use GF soy sauce and noodles*

PER SERVING:
143 KCAL
7.6G CARBS

low-calorie cooking spray
2 garlic cloves, peeled and
    thinly sliced
2.5cm (1in) piece of root ginger,
    peeled and sliced into fine strips
1 red chilli, deseeded and
    finely sliced
200g Tenderstem broccoli
300g broccoli, cut into florets
350g cooked king prawns
2 tbsp light soy sauce
1 tsp granulated sweetener
½ tsp Chinese 5-spice
sea salt and freshly ground
    black pepper

TO ACCOMPANY *(optional)*
4 nests of egg noodles, cooked
    according to packet instructions
    (+ 129 kcal per serving)

Place a large wok or frying pan on a high heat. Spray with low-calorie cooking spray and add the garlic, ginger and chilli. Stir-fry for 2 minutes, moving the ingredients around the pan to stop them from burning.

Add the Tenderstem broccoli and broccoli florets to the wok and combine with the garlic, ginger and chilli. Keep on a high heat and add 3 tablespoons of water. Cook the broccoli for 5 minutes, stirring frequently, until the broccoli is almost tender but still has bite.

Add the remaining ingredients, season with salt and pepper to taste and mix well. Cook for another 5 minutes until the prawns are heated through thoroughly.

Serve immediately on its own, or with the noodles or your choice of accompaniment.

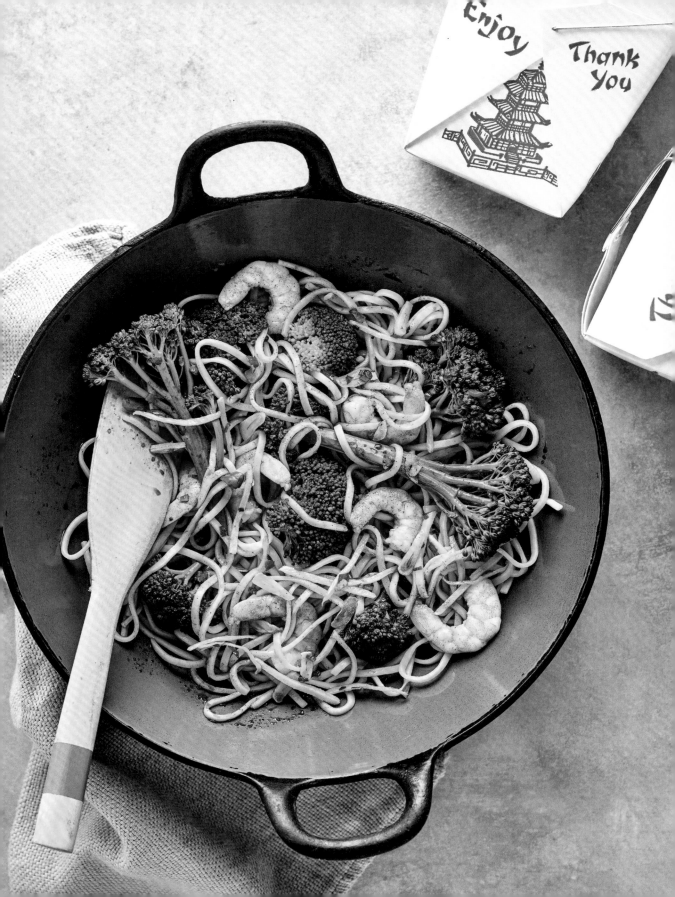

ASIAN PORK MEATBALLS

🕐 **5 MINS** | 🍲 **30 MINS** | ✕ **SERVES 4**

Meatballs are a great, tasty and filling way to get your protein fix. Add a bit of Asian spicing and some spiced ketchup for a tasty little bite that can either be served with a side salad for a light meal, or on its own as a flavourful snack.

F **GF**

→ use a GF stock cube, soy and relish

PER SERVING:
272 KCAL
12G CARBS

500g 5%-fat pork mince
1 courgette, peeled and grated
1 carrot, peeled and grated
4 spring onions, trimmed and
    finely chopped
1 medium egg, beaten
1 tbsp garlic granules
1 tsp onion granules
½ tsp Chinese 5-spice
1 pork stock cube
low-calorie cooking spray
4 tbsp soy sauce
2 tsp Worcestershire sauce
    or Henderson's relish
1 tsp lime juice
sea salt and freshly ground
    black pepper

**FOR THE CHAR SIU
KETCHUP**
250g passata
1 tbsp tomato puree
2 tbsp dark soy sauce
2 tsp Worcestershire sauce
1 tsp lime juice
1 tsp garlic granules
1 tsp granulated sweetener
½ tsp Chinese 5-spice

Preheat the oven to 220°C (fan 200°C/gas mark 7).

Put the pork mince, courgette, carrot and spring onions into a large bowl. Add the egg, garlic granules, onion granules and Chinese 5-spice and crumble in the pork stock cube. Mix well with clean hands until combined, then shape the pork mix into 16–20 x 2cm (¾ in) diameter balls. (You can freeze them at this point if you like – defrost fully before cooking.)

Spray a large frying pan with low-calorie cooking spray and place over a medium heat. You will need to cook the meatballs in two batches. When the pan has heated up, carefully place half the meatballs into it and spray the tops with some more low-calorie cooking spray. Fry for 5 minutes before gently turning them and frying for a further 5 minutes. The meatballs will be fragile until cooked through, so try not to touch them for the first 5 minutes as they are most likely to break apart at this point. If it seems like they are sticking, reduce the heat and add a splash of water to the pan. After another minute carefully try again.

When the outside is cooked, the meat will have turned white and the meatballs will be firmer. Once the first batch is ready, place the meatballs in a large roasting dish. Repeat the process with the second batch. When these are cooked, place them in the roasting dish with the first batch and pour over the soy sauce, Worcestershire sauce and lime juice and season with salt and pepper. Place the roasting dish in the oven and cook for a further 10 minutes. When the meatballs are ready, any liquid will have reduced, and they will be a darker brown colour and much firmer. (At this point, you could allow the meatballs to cool and freeze in an airtight container for reheating on another day.)

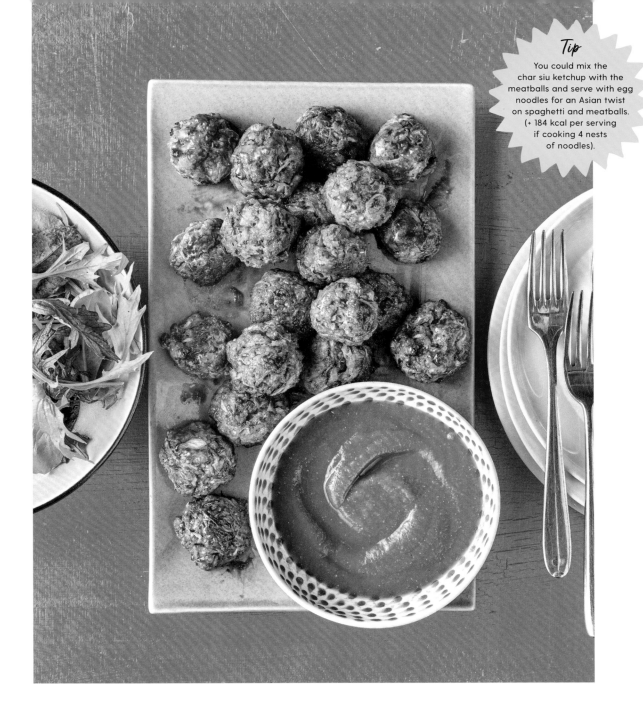

Tip

You could mix the char siu ketchup with the meatballs and serve with egg noodles for an Asian twist on spaghetti and meatballs. (+ 184 kcal per serving if cooking 4 nests of noodles).

TO ACCOMPANY *(optional)*

75g mixed side salad
(+ 15 kcal per serving)

Meanwhile, add the ketchup ingredients to a small saucepan, season with salt and pepper and simmer over a medium–low heat for 10 minutes until thickened. Remove the meatballs from the oven and serve with the ketchup for dipping. (The sauce can also be allowed to cool and frozen separately.)

CHICKEN *and* ASPARAGUS QUICHE

⏱ **5 MINS** | 🍲 **32 MINS** | ✗ **SERVES 6**

Quiche is definitely a party staple, and this chicken and asparagus version offers a protein-filled light dish to take to your next celebration. Quark is a great low-calorie alternative to heavier creams or yoghurts, and omitting the crust from this recipe means that each slice comes in at only 192 calories.

F GF

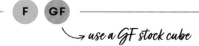

→ *use a GF stock cube*

PER SERVING:
192 KCAL
4.3G CARBS

1 chicken breast (skin and visible fat removed), cut into 1cm (½ in) chunks

1 large onion, peeled and finely chopped

low-calorie cooking spray

100ml chicken stock (1 chicken stock cube dissolved in 100ml boiling water)

sea salt and freshly ground black pepper

8 eggs

2 tbsp quark

60g reduced-fat Cheddar, finely grated

125g asparagus spears, trimmed and cut into 1cm (½ in) pieces

Preheat the oven to 200°C (fan 180°C/gas mark 6).

Put the chicken and onion in a frying pan and spray with some low-calorie cooking spray. Gently sauté over a medium heat for 2 minutes, until the chicken is white on the outside. It won't be cooked fully, only the outside will be coloured.

Add the stock to the pan and simmer for 5 minutes, until the onions are soft, the chicken is cooked through and there is no liquid left in the pan. Season with salt and pepper.

Beat the eggs and quark together in a bowl until smooth, add half the grated cheese and season with salt and pepper. Add the chicken, onion and asparagus to a roughly 23cm (9in) flan dish. Pour over the egg mixture. Sprinkle the other half of the grated cheese on top. Place the dish in the centre of the oven for 25 minutes, or until the quiche has set all the way through and is golden on top.

Remove from the oven and serve hot or cold. You can also cover and freeze for another day once cooled.

MAKE *it* VEGGIE

Use a chicken substitute or double the quantity of asparagus, and swap the chicken stock for vegetable stock.

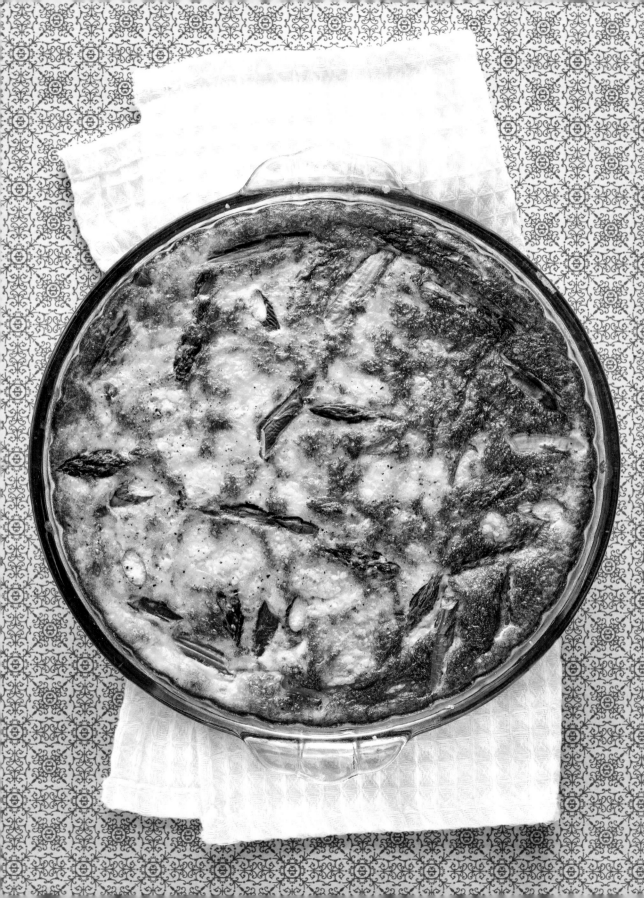

QUESADILLA

⏱ **5 MINS** | 🍲 **15 MINS** | ✕ **SERVES 4**

This recipe is based on the traditional Mexican dish. We've packed low-calorie tortilla wraps with melted cheese, beans and a spicy sauce, but we've cut out all the oils and toasted them in low-calorie cooking spray to crisp them up for the perfect sharing plate. We've served it with a simple tomato salsa which helps to cool some of the fire in the chilli sauce!

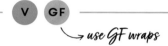

V GF

↳ use GF wraps

PER SERVING:
252 KCAL
32G CARBS

1 x 290g tin mixed beans in
    chilli sauce
½ yellow pepper, deseeded
    and diced
sea salt and finely ground
    black pepper
1 large tomato, finely chopped
2 tbsp chopped fresh coriander
½ small red onion, peeled
    and finely diced
1 tsp red wine vinegar
4 low-calorie tortilla wraps
160g grated reduced-fat
    mozzarella

TO ACCOMPANY *(optional)*
Barbecue Potato Wedges,
    page 214 (+ 141 kcal per serving)

Add the mixed beans in chilli sauce to a frying pan with the diced yellow pepper. Season with salt and pepper and cook over a medium heat for 10 minutes until the sauce has reduced.

While the beans are reducing, make the salsa by placing the tomato, coriander, red onion and red wine vinegar in a small bowl and mix. Season with a little salt.

Remove the beans from the frying pan and wipe the pan clean. Place the frying pan back on a medium heat and add one of the tortilla wraps to the dry pan. Top the wrap with half of the bean mixture, spreading it evenly over the wrap. Sprinkle over half of the mozzarella and top with a few teaspoons of the tomato salsa. Place a second tortilla wrap on top, and once the bottom wrap has just started to colour, carefully flip the quesadilla over with a fish slice or spatula. Leave for 2 minutes to crisp the bottom, remove from the frying pan and cut into quarters.

Repeat the process to make the second quesadilla. Serve with the remaining salsa.

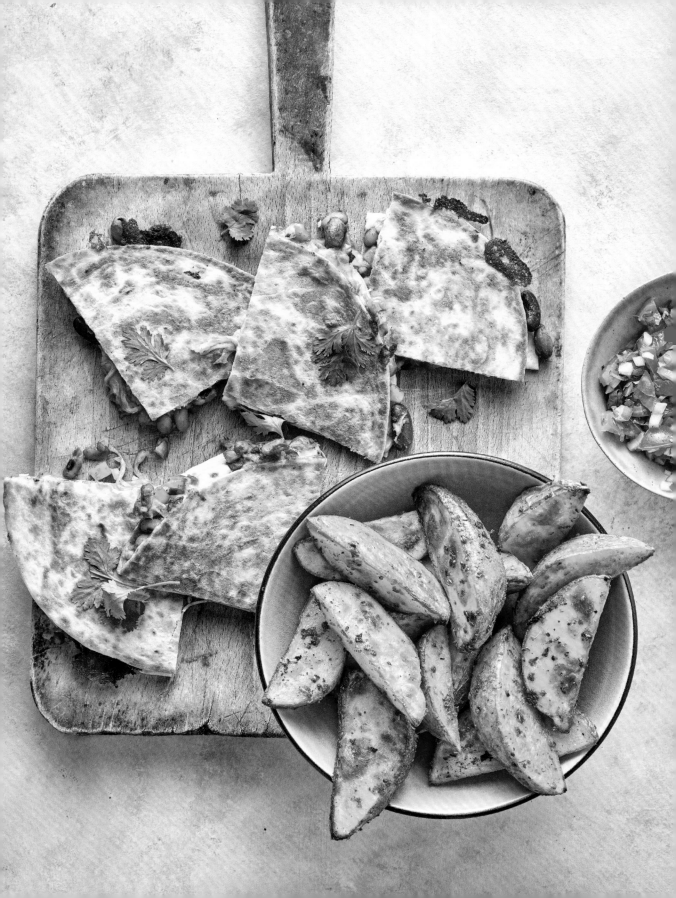

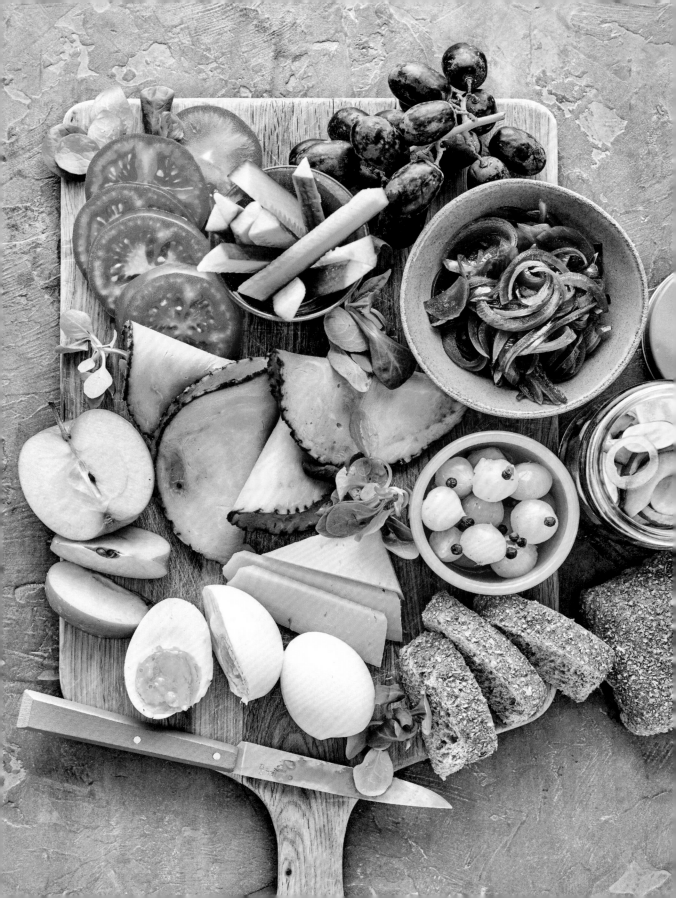

PLOUGHMAN'S PLATTER
with HOMEMADE CHUTNEY

🕐 **5 MINS** | 🍲 **30 MINS** | ✕ **SERVES 2**

Our version of a ploughman's lunch combines filling vegetables and salad with some reduced-fat Cheddar and wholemeal bread. Bring it together with our sweet and tangy red onion chutney which can be whipped up in just 30 minutes!

PER SERVING:
382 KCAL
43.9G CARBS

FOR THE CHUTNEY
2 small red onions, peeled and
    thinly sliced
4 tbsp balsamic vinegar
1 tsp Worcestershire sauce or
    Henderson's relish
1 tbsp granulated sweetener
200ml water
sea salt and freshly ground
    black pepper

FOR THE PLATTER
2 eggs
sea salt and freshly ground
    black pepper
40g reduced-fat mature Cheddar
4 thin slices of lean ham
2 x 45g wholemeal rolls, sliced
16 small silverskin pickled onions,
    drained (or serve with Quickles,
    see page 244)
160g cucumber, cut into sticks
6 radishes, sliced in half
1 tomato, sliced
1 apple, sliced (about 75g)
20 grapes
handful of lamb's lettuce

Place all the chutney ingredients in a saucepan, with a pinch each of salt and pepper. Bring to the boil, then reduce the heat to low, cover and simmer with the lid on for 15 minutes. Remove the lid and cook for a further 15 minutes, or until the liquid has reduced and the onions are soft, dark and sticky. Remove from the heat and leave to cool.

While the chutney is cooking, add the eggs to another saucepan. Cover with water and bring to the boil. Once the water is bubbling, cook for 6 minutes. Remove the eggs from the pan with a slotted spoon and leave to cool in a bowl of cold water.

Once the eggs are cooled, peel them carefully. You can do this under a running tap to make it easier. Slice in half and season with salt and pepper.

Arrange the chutney, eggs, cheese, ham, bread, onions, cucumber, radishes, tomato, apple, grapes and lettuce on a board and serve.

LEMON *and* PEPPER
CHICKEN TAGLIATELLE

🕐 **5 MINS** (PLUS MARINATING TIME) | 🍲 **15–20 MINS** | ✕ **SERVES 4**

This dish is beautifully simple, but don't let the sparse ingredient list fool you: this dish is full of flavour. Tagliatelle is a really versatile pasta, going well with thick sauces as well as basic elements such as tomatoes or, in this case, lemon juice. Marinating the chicken in the lemon and pepper is a really important step, so don't skip this; we promise you won't regret it!

PER SERVING:
397 KCAL
35G CARBS

2 lemons
freshly ground black pepper
4 chicken breasts, about
    165g each (skin and visible
    fat removed)
sea salt
low-calorie cooking spray
200g tagliatelle
2 egg yolks
a pinch of chopped fresh chives
    or parsley, to serve (optional)

Halve and squeeze one of the lemons into a bowl and add ¼–½ teaspoon of black pepper according to your taste. Place the chicken breasts in the bowl and mix well. Allow to marinate for 30 minutes.

Remove the chicken and season with salt. Spray a griddle pan or heavy-based frying pan with low-calorie cooking spray and place over a medium heat. Add the chicken breasts to the pan and cook for 14–15 minutes, turning halfway through. Ensure the chicken is cooked through, with no pink remaining.

Meanwhile, bring a large pan of salted water to the boil and cook the tagliatelle, according to packet instructions – usually 9–10 minutes.

Mix the egg yolks with the juice of the remaining lemon and add a little salt and pepper.

When the pasta is cooked, drain in a colander, reserving a little of the cooking water, and return the pasta to the pan. While still hot, stir in the egg and lemon juice. The heat of the pasta will cook the egg. Add a little of the reserved pasta water if you wish.

Divide the pasta between four plates and slice the chicken breasts, placing one on top of each plate. Scatter with fresh chives or parsley, if you wish.

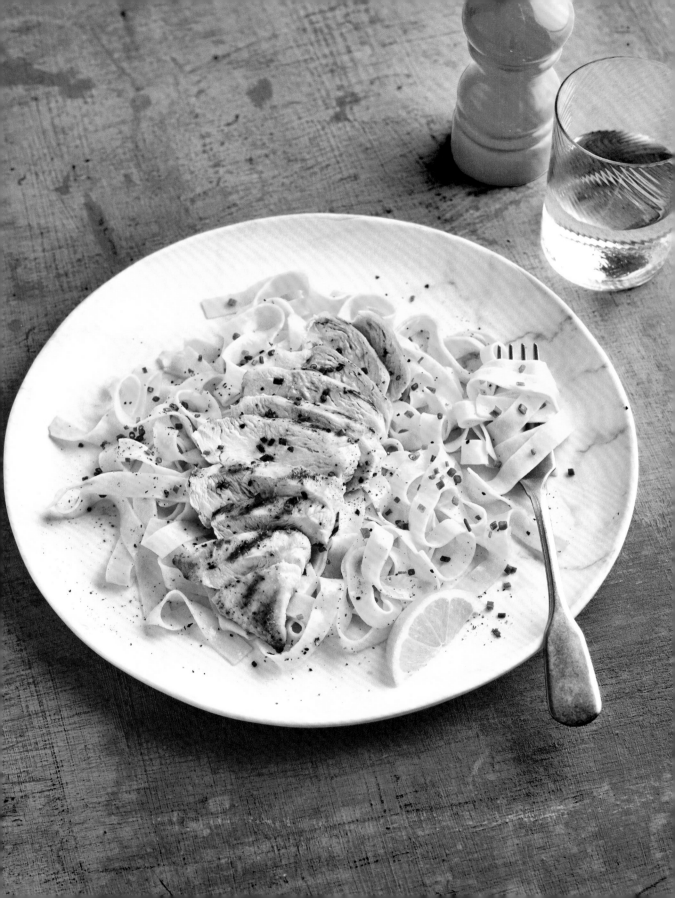

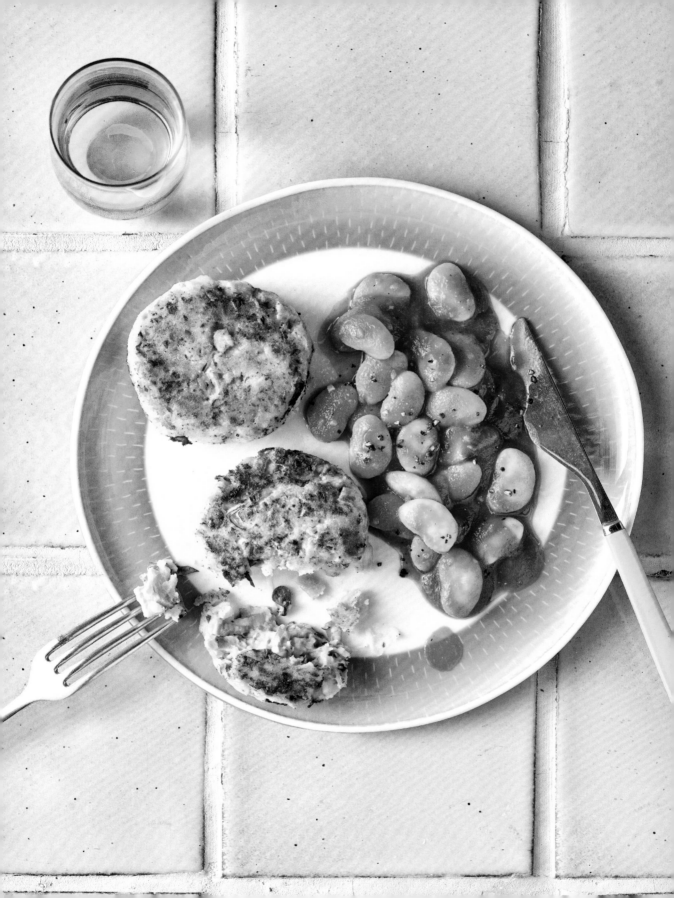

HAM *and* POTATO CAKES

🕐 **10 MINS** | 🍲 **30 MINS** | ✕ **SERVES 4**

These ham and potato cakes taste just as good as the deep-fried versions, but without the need for all the oil and calories. The mustard adds a real depth of flavour and a sprinkle of seasoning makes them proper yum! So simple and delicious, they make a great midweek meal for all the family to enjoy.

PER SERVING:
259 KCAL
33G CARBS

700g potatoes, peeled
   and chopped
300g cooked ham
4 spring onions, trimmed
   and sliced
1 tsp mustard powder
2 tsp chopped fresh parsley
sea salt and freshly ground
   black pepper
1 large egg yolk, beaten
low-calorie cooking spray

TO ACCOMPANY *(optional)*
Giant Baked Beans, page 36
   (+ 144 kcal per serving)

Cook the potatoes in a large pan of boiling salted water for 20–30 minutes, until a knife slides easily into the potatoes. Drain thoroughly and allow them to dry for a minute or two. Place in a bowl and mash well.

Finely chop the ham and add to the potatoes, along with the spring onions, mustard powder and chopped parsley. Mix well. Season with salt and pepper to taste. Add the egg yolk, a little at a time – this will help to bind the mixture. Mix well, then form into eight equal-sized cakes.

Spray a frying pan with low-calorie cooking spray and place over a medium heat. Place four cakes in the pan and cook for about 5 minutes until the bottom is a golden brown. Gently flip them over, being careful not to break them up, and cook for a further 5 minutes. If you think they are browning too quickly, reduce the heat.

Slide onto a plate and keep warm while you cook the remaining four ham and potato cakes. Serve two cakes per person, with a green salad or some baked beans.

Tip

These cakes are a bit fragile, so don't be tempted to keep flipping or lifting them out of the pan. Gently turn them over once to reduce the risk of them falling apart.

SAUSAGE *and* ONION PLAIT

🕐 **15 MINS** | 🍲 **30–40 MINS** | ✕ **SERVES 6**

These plaits are a great alternative to a pasty or a pie, and by using a low-calorie tortilla wrap, the calorie count is so much lower than your standard greasy pastry. Seasoning the pork mince thoroughly is key to making these the tasty treats that we all deserve!

F

PER SERVING:
268 KCAL
27G CARBS

2 red onions, peeled
100ml stock (1 pork or chicken
    stock cube dissolved in
    100ml boiling water)
1 tbsp Worcestershire sauce
    or Henderson's relish
3 tbsp balsamic vinegar
500g 5%-fat pork mince
1 tsp garlic granules
½ tsp dried sage
½ tsp dried rosemary
½ tsp mustard powder
sea salt and freshly ground
    black pepper
6 low-calorie tortilla wraps
1 egg
low-calorie cooking spray

TO ACCOMPANY *(optional)*
Ketchup Tomatoes, page 221
    (+ 38 kcal per serving)

Tip
If you are struggling
with the plait, just fold the
wraps up like a parcel
or roll them up like a fat
sausage roll. They'll still
taste great!

Preheat oven to 200°C (fan 180°C/gas mark 6).

Thinly slice the onions and add to a frying pan with the stock, Worcestershire sauce and balsamic vinegar. Place over a low–medium heat and simmer for around 5 minutes until the onions are soft and starting to brown and the liquid has reduced.

While the onions are cooking, mix the pork mince in a bowl with the garlic granules, sage, rosemary, mustard powder and salt and pepper. When the onions are done, mix them into the pork mince.

This is a bit of a tricky technique but you can use the images on pages 102–3 to help you. Take a wrap and fold it into three equal sections. Press firmly so you can see the marks when you unfold it. Open out the wrap and fold it in half. When you do this you should be able to see the marks you made earlier. Using a sharp knife, make a cut from the line to the edge of the wrap. Measure a finger's width and make another cut at the same angle. Continue all the way up the side of the folded wrap. Unfold the wrap.

Brush the whole wrap with beaten egg, paying extra attention to the edges. Place a sixth of the pork mix across the wrap, adding it to the centre and gently patting down into a flat sausage shape. Fold the top and bottom of the wrap in, then, starting at the end closest to you, fold the bottom-left strip up towards the top right-hand corner of the wrap. Fold the bottom-right strip over towards the top-left corner of the wrap. Fold the bottom-right strip over towards the top-left corner of the wrap. Alternate the remaining strips until all the filling is enclosed. Repeat with the remaining wraps and mince.

Continued...

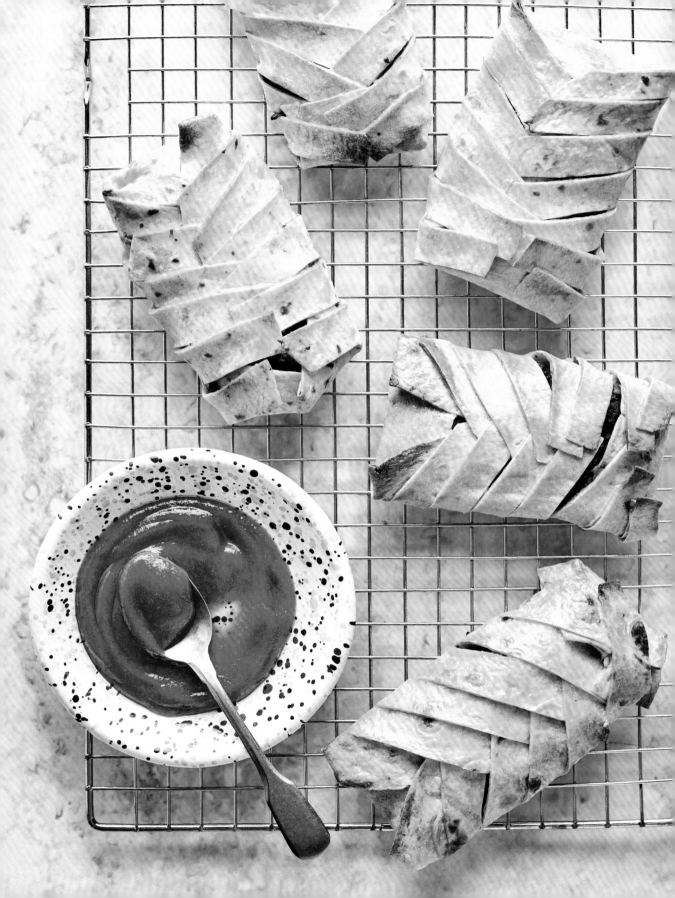

Continued...

Line a baking tray with foil and spray liberally with the low-calorie cooking spray. Place the plaits onto the tray, plait side down. Beat the egg and brush over the side of the wrap facing up. Spray the wraps with low-calorie cooking spray and put the tray into the middle of the preheated oven for 15–20 minutes. They should be golden and a little firm once done. Turn them over and brush the plait side with the egg. Spray with low-calorie cooking spray again and put them back in the oven for another 15–20 minutes.

When they are ready they will be crispy and golden brown. These can also be frozen once cooled. Make sure you defrost thoroughly before reheating them.

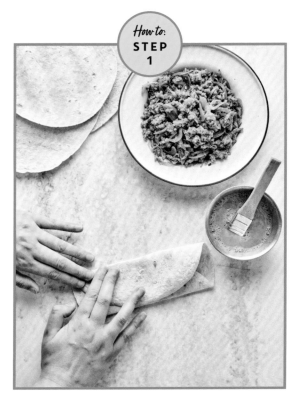

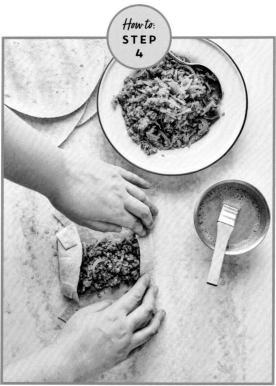

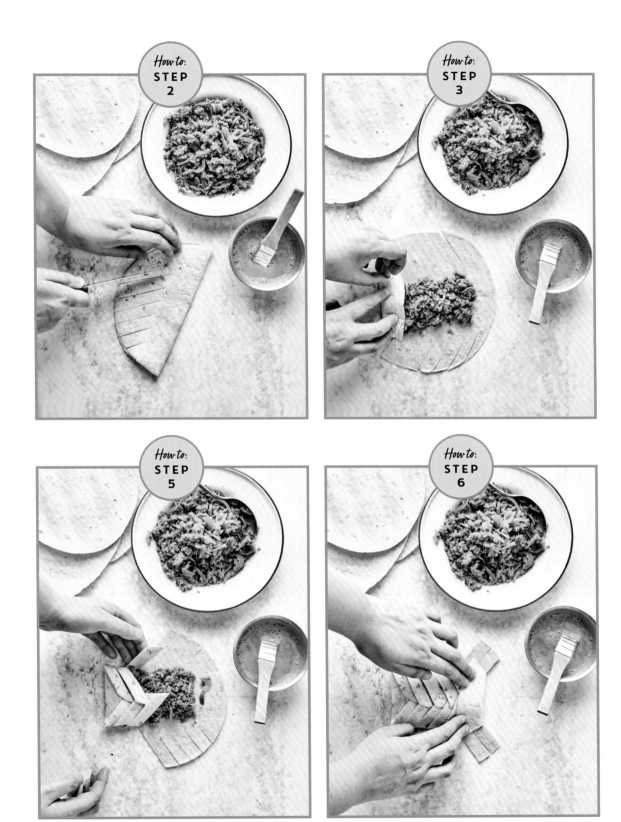

How to:
STEP 2

How to:
STEP 3

How to:
STEP 5

How to:
STEP 6

QUICK MEALS

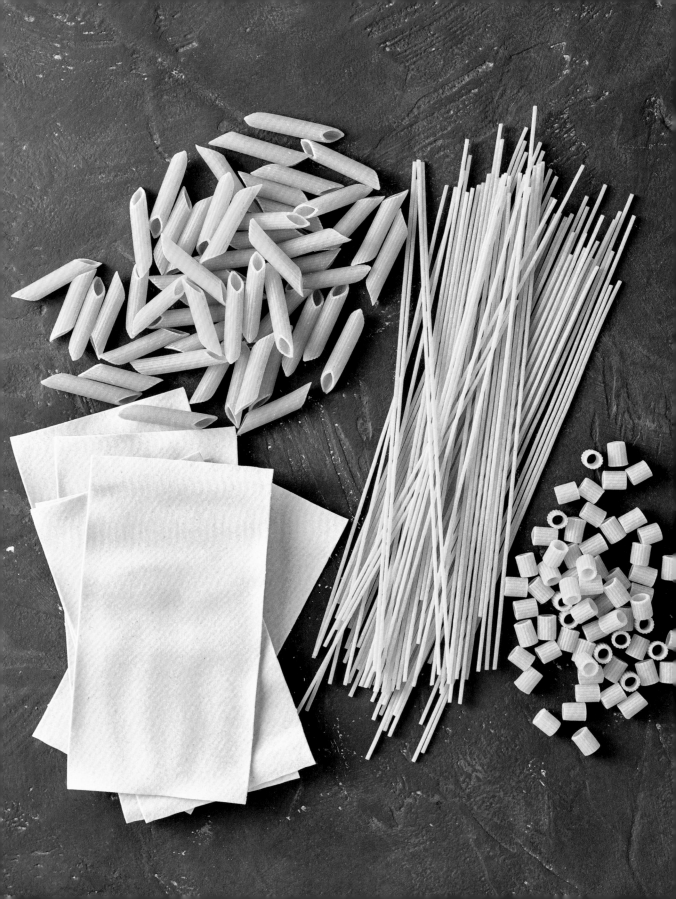

The QUESADILLA *is* UTTERLY DELICIOUS

JACKIE

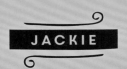

LEMON + PEPPER CHICKEN TAGLIATELLE was *demolished* with praise and requests to make it again

ANITA

TANDOORI SALMON WITH MANGO SALSA will *definitely* be a regular dish in our house

JIM

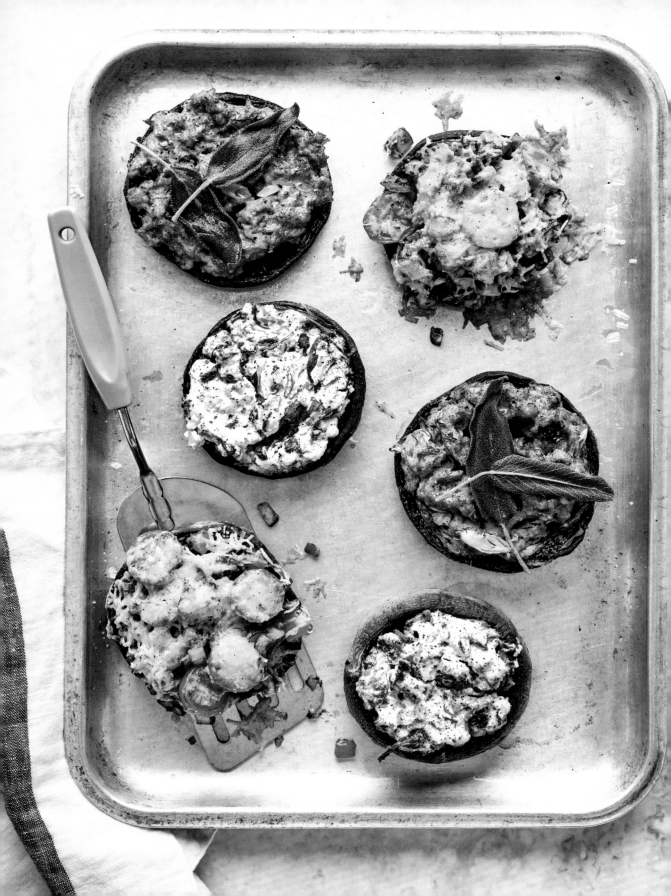

STUFFED MUSHROOMS

🕐 **10 MINS** | 🍲 **10–12 MINS** | ✗ **SERVES 2**

Stuffed mushrooms make a great starter or a side, or even a meal with some salad leaves, and there are so many combinations to play with. Portobello mushrooms are so great for anybody looking to cut calories, plus they are low-carb, rich in antioxidants and add flavour. We've pulled together our top three recipes to share with you.

V   GF

PER SERVING:
74 KCAL
3.9G CARBS

2 large flat mushrooms,
   such as portobello
low-calorie cooking spray
1 spring onion, trimmed and
   finely chopped
25g spinach
45g ricotta
sea salt and finely ground
   black pepper

SPINACH AND RICOTTA

Preheat the oven to 200°C (fan 180°C/gas mark 6).

Remove the stalks from the mushrooms and dice them finely, then place them back into the middle of the mushrooms.

Spray a frying pan with some low-calorie cooking spray, then sauté the spring onion until softened, but not coloured. Toss the spinach in with the spring onion and continue to cook until it has wilted, then remove from the heat and drain off any excess moisture. Mix in the ricotta and season with a little salt and pepper.

Spoon the mixture into the mushrooms and place them on a baking tray.

Cook in the oven for 10–12 minutes, or until the mushrooms are cooked.

Continued...

Continued...

MEDITERRANEAN VEGETABLE

PER SERVING:
152 KCAL
9.4G CARBS

2 large flat mushrooms,
   such as portobello
low-calorie cooking spray
30g peeled red onion, diced
60g courgette, diced
½ red pepper, deseeded and diced
1 tsp tomato puree
pinch of dried Italian herbs
1 tsp balsamic vinegar
sea salt and freshly ground
   black pepper
4 cherry tomatoes, cut in half
35g vegetarian Italian hard
   cheese, grated

TO ACCOMPANY *(optional)*
75g mixed side salad
   (+ 15 kcal)

Preheat the oven to 200°C (fan 180°C/gas mark 6).

Remove the stalks from the mushrooms and dice them finely.

Spray a frying pan with some low-calorie cooking spray, then sauté the onion, courgette, pepper and mushroom stalks over a medium heat until they are cooked. This should take around 5–6 minutes. Add the tomato puree, herbs and balsamic vinegar, stir well and season to taste with salt and pepper.

Spoon the mixture into the mushrooms, put 2 tomato halves on top of each and place them on a baking tray.

Divide the Italian hard cheese equally between the two mushrooms and sprinkle over the top.

Cook in the oven for 10–12 minutes until the mushrooms are cooked and the cheese is golden brown.

PORK, SAGE AND ONION

PER SERVING:
54 KCAL
2.4G CARBS

2 large flat mushrooms,
   such as portobello
50g lean pork mince
1 spring onion, trimmed and
   finely chopped
½ tsp sage, dried or chopped
   fresh, plus extra whole leaves
   to garnish (optional)
sea salt and freshly ground
   black pepper

Preheat the oven to 200°C (fan 180°C/gas mark 6).

Remove the stalks from the mushrooms and dice them finely, then place them back into the middle of the mushrooms.

Place the pork mince in a bowl, then add the spring onion, sage and a little salt and pepper. Mix well. Spoon the mixture into the mushrooms and place them on a baking tray.

Cook in the oven for 10–12 minutes, or until the mushrooms and pork are cooked. Serve garnished with sage leaves (if using).

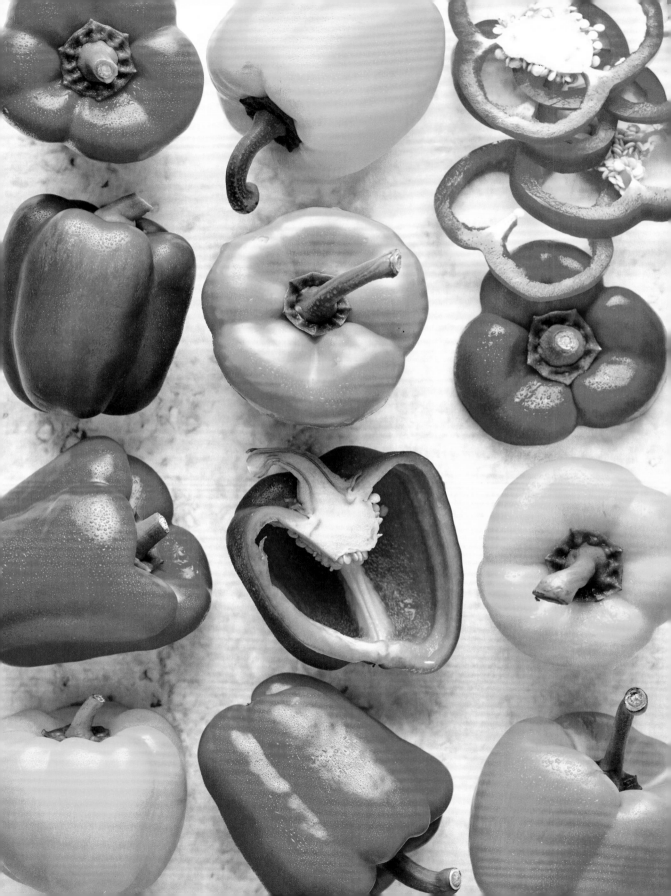

TANDOORI SALMON *with* MANGO SALSA

🕐 **10 MINS** (PLUS MARINATING TIME) | 🍲 **12–15 MINS** | ✕ **SERVES 4**

Salmon is such a versatile fish, and this recipe is great for adding a touch of sophistication to a midweek meal. It tastes and looks amazing, but is so easy to pull together. The spices from the marinated fish, plus the sweetness from the mango dip, make it a flavour sensation.

 GF

PER SERVING:
355 KCAL
13G CARBS

4 x 120g salmon fillets,
   skins removed

FOR THE MARINADE
5 tbsp fat-free natural yoghurt
2 tsp paprika
1 tsp garlic granules
½ tsp ground coriander
½ tsp ground cumin
½ tsp granulated sweetener
squeeze of lime juice

FOR THE SALSA
1 ripe mango, peeled and cut into
   5mm (¼ in) dice
1 red pepper, deseeded and cut
   into 5mm (¼ in) dice
2 spring onions, trimmed and
   thinly sliced
10g fresh coriander, chopped
juice of ½ lime
sea salt and freshly ground
   black pepper

TO ACCOMPANY *(optional)*
80g steamed veg (+ 38 kcal
   per serving)

Preheat the oven to 200°C (fan 180°C/gas mark 6).

Mix together the yoghurt, spices and squeeze of lime juice. Coat the salmon fillets in the marinade, cover and leave for 30 minutes.

Mix together the mango, red pepper and spring onions in a bowl together with the chopped coriander and the lime juice. Season with salt and pepper.

Place the salmon on a baking sheet and cook for 15 minutes. Serve topped with the salsa.

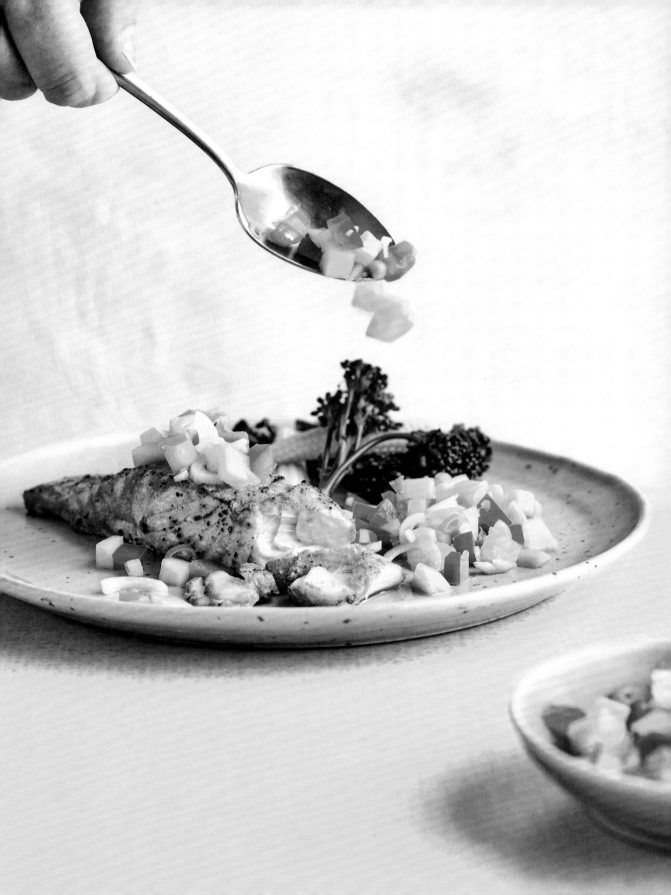

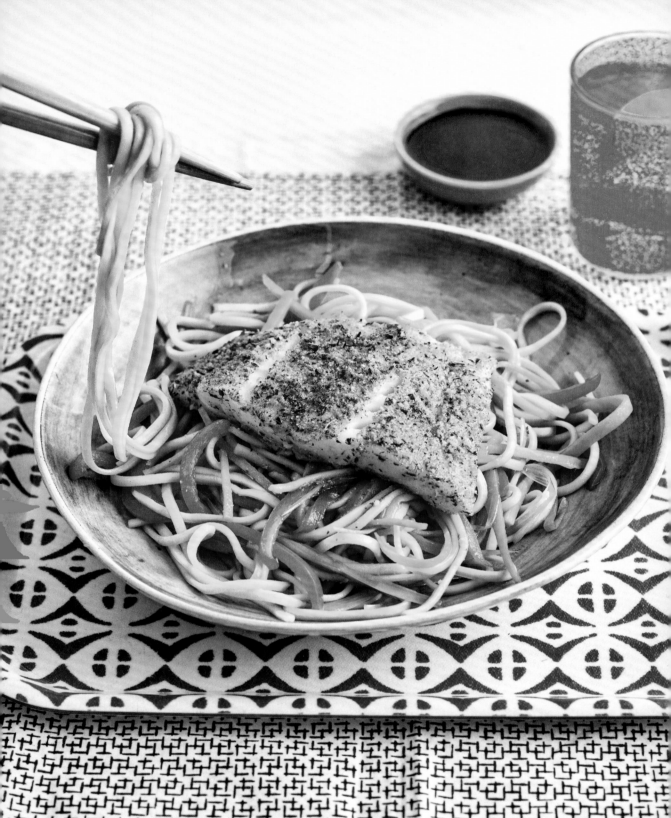

THAI-SPICED FISH
with NOODLES

🕐 **10 MINS** | 🍲 **15 MINS** | ✕ **SERVES 4**

Ready in only 25 minutes, this dish is bursting with flavour from the spice mix. You can use almost any white fish for this recipe; we recommend cod or hake. White fish is really great for adding a protein fix, with the added benefit of being low-fat.

→ use a GF noodles and soy sauce

PER SERVING:
340 KCAL
41G CARBS

4 cod or hake fillets (about 150g each)
sea salt
low-calorie cooking spray
4 noodle nests (about 200g)
1 red or yellow pepper, deseeded and cut into strips
4 spring onions, trimmed and thinly sliced lengthways
1 medium carrot, peeled and cut into thin strips (julienne)
3 tbsp light soy sauce
juice of 1 lemon
10g fresh coriander, chopped

FOR THE SPICE MIX
1 tsp ground cumin
1 tsp garlic granules
1 tsp onion granules
1 tsp dried mint
¼ tsp chilli powder (mild or hot, depending on your preference)
¼ tsp ground ginger
zest of 1 lemon
pinch of sea salt

Preheat the oven to 200°C (fan 180°C/gas mark 6).

Mix all the spice mix ingredients together.

Pat the fish dry using some kitchen towel, then sprinkle with a little salt. Coat the fish, on both sides, with the spice mix and place the fillets on a baking tray that has been sprayed with some low-calorie cooking spray.

Cook in the oven for about 10–15 minutes, until the fish is opaque.

While the fish is cooking, place the noodles in a pan of boiling water, and cook according to the packet instructions. This usually takes around 4–6 minutes. Drain the noodles and allow them to cool in some cold water. This will stop them sticking together.

Spray a wok or large frying pan with some low-calorie cooking spray, then, over a medium–high heat, add the pepper, spring onions and carrot. Cook for 4–5 minutes until they are just cooked, but still quite crunchy.

Drain the noodles and add to the pan, along with the soy sauce and lemon juice. Cook for a minute or two, until the noodles are hot and well coated. Stir in the coriander and divide the noodles equally between four plates.

Remove the fish from the oven, place one piece of fish on top of each plate of noodles and serve.

WARM GREEN BEAN
and FETA SALAD

🕐 **5 MINS** | 🍲 **10–12 MINS** | ✕ **SERVES 4**

This recipe is quick and easy to throw together. The salty feta combined with the sweet pepper and the acidity from the lemon juice gives it the most amazing flavour, plus you can add some heat with the chilli flakes. At only 111 calories per serving, you can enjoy this on its own as a light lunch or as a side to your main evening meal.

use a veggie cheese ⤶

PER SERVING:
111 KCAL
6.9G CARBS

low-calorie cooking spray
240g green beans, washed
    and trimmed
1 small red onion, peeled, cut in
    half and sliced
1 medium red pepper, deseeded
    and sliced
1 garlic clove, peeled and
    finely chopped
pinch of dried chilli flakes (you
    can use more if you like it spicy)
sea salt and freshly ground
    black pepper
2 tbsp water
juice of 1 lemon, plus extra
    wedges to serve
130g reduced-fat feta or Greek-
    style salad cheese, crumbled

Spray a wok or frying pan with some low-calorie cooking spray and sauté the green beans and onion over a medium heat for about 3 minutes. Add the pepper, garlic and chilli flakes. Season with some salt and pepper, stir and cook for another minute.

Add the water, stir and continue cooking for another 5–6 minutes or until the beans are almost cooked (they should still have a bit of bite, but you can cook them for a few more minutes if you prefer them more well done).

Add the lemon juice and cook for another minute. Stir in the crumbled feta, taste to check the seasoning and serve.

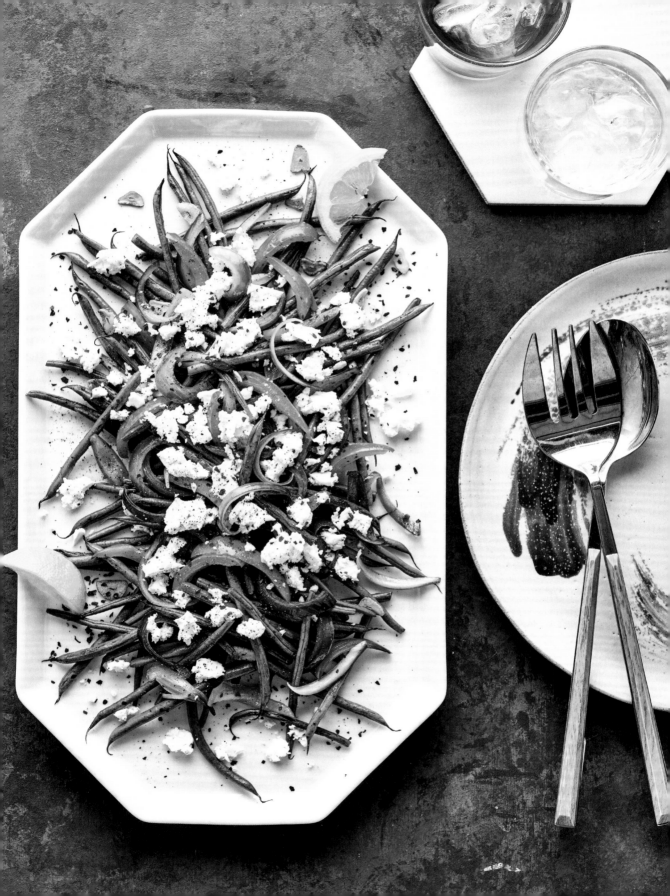

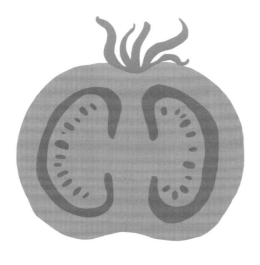

BATCH
COOK

THAI CHICKEN CAKES

🕐 **15 MINS** | 🍲 **10 MINS** | ✗ **SERVES 4**

Thai fishcakes may be the norm, but this chicken version is just as tasty. The recipe uses water chestnuts, which, despite the name, aren't actually nuts! They are a great source of fibre and are low in calories, making them perfect for this dish. Served with a dipping sauce, these are a great starter before serving our Thai-spiced Fish with Noodles (see page 113). To save time, substitute chicken or turkey mince for the chicken breast.

 F **GF**

PER SERVING:
198 KCAL
6G CARBS

1 x 225g tin water chestnuts, drained
4 spring onions, trimmed and thinly sliced
zest and ½ juice of 1 lime, plus extra wedges to serve (optional)
2 garlic cloves, peeled and minced or grated
1cm (½in) piece of root ginger, peeled and grated
10g fresh coriander, chopped
1 tsp dried chilli flakes (or to taste)
2 tsp plus 2 tbsp light soy sauce
4 chicken breasts, about 600g (skin and visible fat removed)
sea salt and freshly ground black pepper
low-calorie cooking spray
½ tsp granulated sweetener

Preheat the oven to 200°C (fan 180°C/gas mark 6). Using a food processor, finely chop the water chestnuts. Place in a mixing bowl with the spring onions, lime zest, garlic, two-thirds of the grated ginger, coriander, chilli flakes and 2 teaspoons of soy sauce.

Cut the chicken into chunks, then mince in the food processor. Add the mince to the bowl and mix all the ingredients together. Check the seasoning by cooking a penny-sized piece in a frying pan with some low-calorie cooking spray. Add salt and pepper to the chicken mix according to taste.

Divide into twenty equal-sized balls, shape into cakes and place on a baking sheet that has been sprayed with low calorie-cooking spray. Cook in the oven for 10 minutes, until the juices run clear and there is no pink in the chicken.

While the chicken is cooking, make the dipping sauce. Mix together the remaining 2 tablespoons of soy sauce, the lime juice, the sweetener and the remaining ginger.

Serve five bite-size cakes per portion with the dipping sauce on the side, and lime wedges (if using).

HOW *to* BATCH

You can freeze these before or after cooking. If freezing raw, defrost thoroughly (preferably in the fridge or microwave on defrost setting) before cooking in the oven. If cooked, allow to cool within 2 hours before freezing. Make sure they are defrosted completely before reheating in the oven. Find detailed guidelines on reheating on page 11.

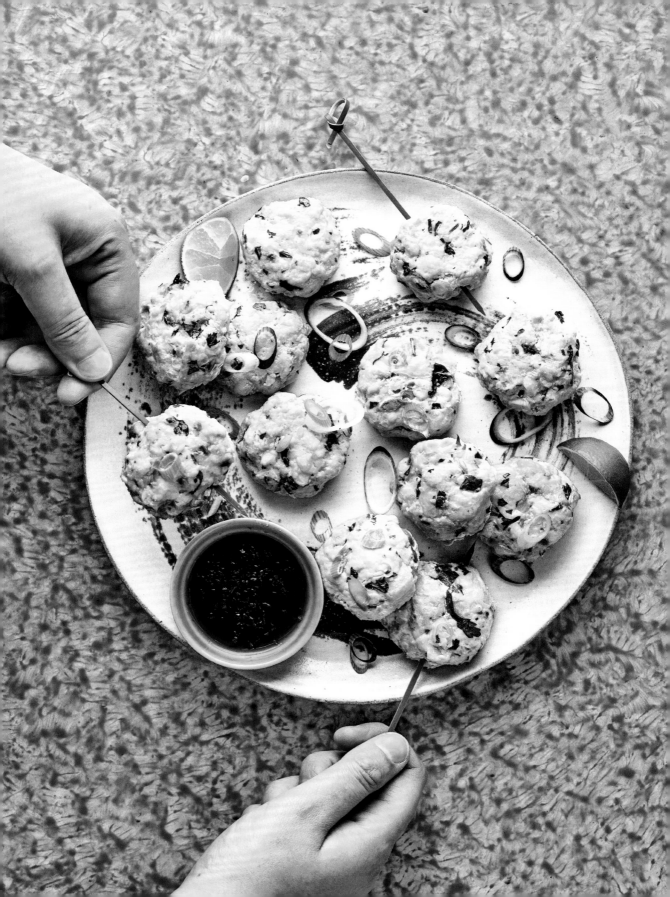

CHIPOTLE TURKEY MEATBALLS

🕐 **15 MINS** | 🗑 **30 MINS** | ✕ **SERVES 4**

These meatballs in a chipotle-spiced sauce are the perfect, simple midweek meal for all the family. The rich, flavourful sauce will make them think you've been slaving over the hob for hours. While the meatballs need assembling, that's as much work as you'll need to do, as the rest is throw-in-the-pan stuff.

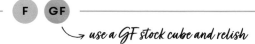

F **GF**

↳ *use a GF stock cube and relish*

PER SERVING:
333 KCAL
34G CARBS

low-calorie cooking spray
1 onion, peeled and chopped
1 carrot, peeled and dices
2 garlic cloves, peeled and minced
2 tsp smoked paprika
½ tsp chipotle chilli flakes
1 x 500g carton passata
300ml chicken stock (1 chicken stock cube dissolved in 300ml boiling water)
2 tbsp Worcestershire sauce or Henderson's relish
sea salt and freshly ground black pepper
200g dried spaghetti

FOR THE MEATBALLS
500g turkey breast mince
1 small onion, peeled and thinly chopped
½ tsp chipotle chilli flakes
1 tsp dried oregano
½ tsp garlic salt
a good grind of black pepper
low-calorie cooking spray

Spray a saucepan with low-calorie cooking spray. Sauté the onion and carrot over a medium heat for 4–5 minutes, until the onion begins to soften. Add the garlic, paprika and chipotle chilli flakes and stir well for another minute. Add the passata, stock and Worcestershire sauce and season with salt and pepper as required. Bring to a gentle simmer, then cover and cook for 20 minutes until the carrots are soft.

Meanwhile, place all the ingredients for the meatballs in a bowl and mix well. Divide into twenty even pieces and roll into balls.

Cook the pasta according to packet instructions.

While the pasta is cooking, spray a frying pan with low-calorie cooking spray and place over a medium–high heat. Add the meatballs and fry on all sides, until sealed and golden. This should take around 10 minutes. Remove the sauce from the heat and blitz with a stick blender, being careful not to splash hot sauce.

Pour the sauce over the meatballs, stir and return to the heat. Simmer for 5–10 minutes and serve.

HOW *to* BATCH

You can freeze the meatballs before or after cooking. If freezing raw, defrost thoroughly (preferably in the fridge or microwave on defrost setting) before frying. You can divide the cooked recipe into individual servings (five meatballs per portion, minus the cooked pasta accompaniment). Allow to cool within 2 hours and freeze. Find detailed guidelines on reheating on page 11.

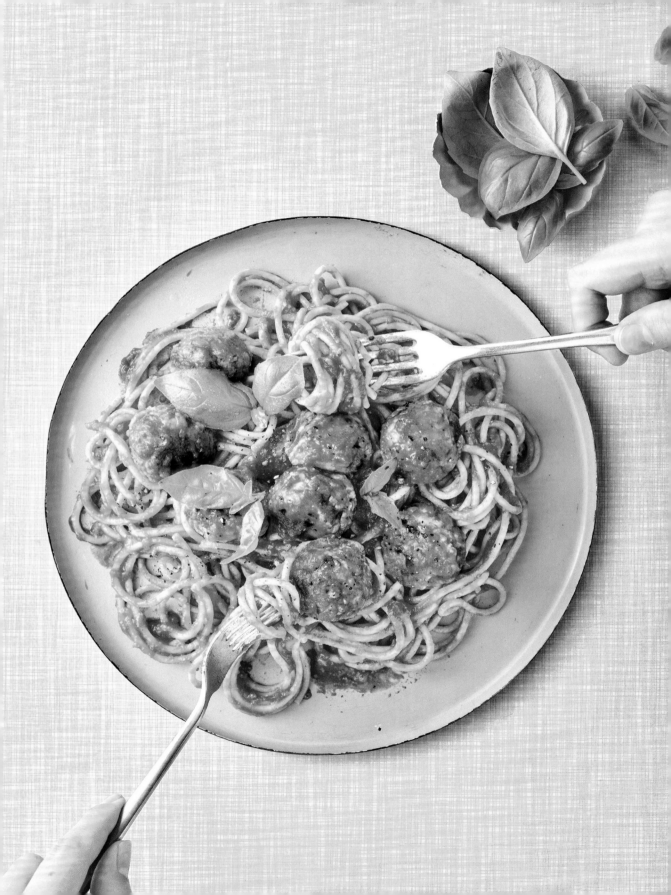

CHEESE *and* ONION CRISPBAKES

🕐 **5 MINS** | 🍲 **45 MINS** | ✕ **SERVES 4**

There aren't very many flavour combinations better than cheese and onion! When combined with some creamy mashed potatoes and given a crispy coating, these simple flavours are transformed into a really comforting and tasty meal – and there's no deep-fat fryer in sight! Serve with a side salad and half a corn on the cob for a full, tasty, cheesy meal for under 400 calories.

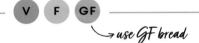

→ *use GF bread*

PER SERVING:
300 KCAL
36G CARBS

500g potatoes, peeled and chopped
120g wholemeal bread
2 medium eggs
80g reduced-fat Cheddar, grated
1 tsp mustard powder
6 spring onions, trimmed and thinly sliced
sea salt and freshly ground black pepper
low-calorie cooking spray

TO ACCOMPANY *(optional)*
Mini corn cob and 75g mixed side salad (+ 47 kcal per serving)

Preheat the oven to 170°C (fan 150°C/gas mark 3). Line a baking tray with greaseproof paper.

Cook the potatoes in a pan of boiling salted water for 20 minutes, until a knife slides easily into the centre of each potato. Drain well, return to the pan and mash.

Using a mini electric chopper or food processor, blitz the wholemeal bread into fine crumbs. Place into a shallow dish. Whisk the eggs in a bowl and set aside.

Add the cheese, mustard powder and spring onions to the mashed potatoes and mix well. Season to taste. Split the mashed potato mix into four. Shape each quarter into a large burger, around 1.5cm (½in) thick. Carefully dip each burger into the egg, and then into the breadcrumbs, coating each side. Place on the baking tray and repeat to make four burgers in total.

Spray each crispbake with low-calorie cooking spray and place in the oven for 25 minutes, turning halfway through the cooking time and spraying again with low-calorie cooking spray. The burgers should be golden and crisp when cooked.

HOW *to* BATCH

Cool within 2 hours of cooking, then freeze the cakes individually. Reheat them from frozen (25–30 minutes at 160°C/fan 140°C/gas mark 3). Find detailed guidelines on reheating on page 11.

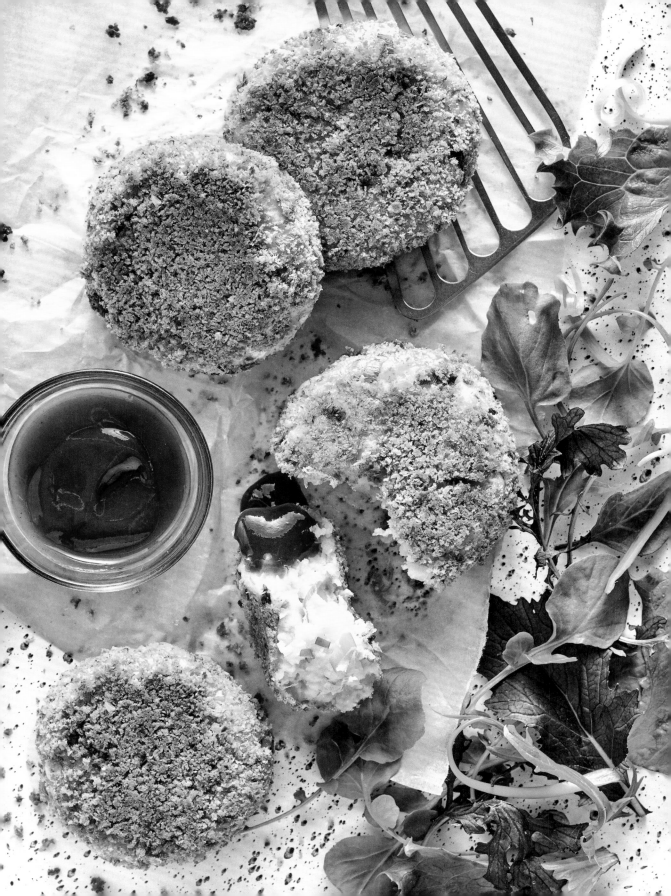

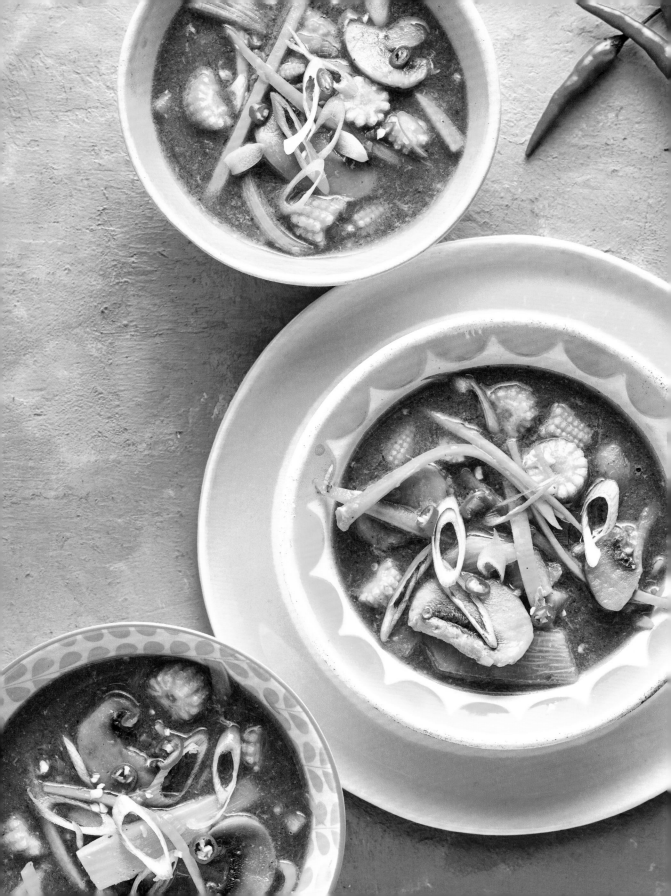

HOT *and* SOUR SOUP

🕐 **10 MINS** | 🍲 **10 MINS** | ✕ **SERVES 4**

This low-cal Hot and Sour Soup packs in the veggies and is the perfect quick meal to prepare on a cold day to warm you up. Xanthan gum is a great ingredient for thickening soup and can be found in most supermarkets in the 'free-from' aisles as a gluten-free variant of cornflour.

V **F** **GF**

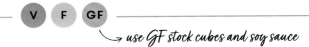
→ *use GF stock cubes and soy sauce*

PER SERVING:
98 KCAL
9G CARBS

low-calorie cooking spray
100g mushrooms, sliced
4 spring onions, trimmed
    and sliced
1 red chilli, deseeded and sliced
2 garlic cloves, peeled and
    minced or grated
1 litre vegetable stock
    (2 vegetable stock cubes
    dissolved in 1 litre boiling water
2 carrots, peeled and cut into
    thin strips (julienne)
75g baby corn, cut into 5mm
    (¼ in)-thick slices
120g tinned bamboo shoots,
    drained
2 tbsp light soy sauce
2 tbsp rice vinegar
½ tsp dried chilli flakes
¼–½ tsp xanthan gum
1 egg

Spray a large saucepan or wok with low-calorie cooking spray. Add the mushrooms, spring onions, sliced chilli and garlic and stir-fry over a medium heat for 3–4 minutes until they are soft. Add the stock, carrots, baby corn, bamboo shoots, soy sauce, vinegar and chilli flakes.

Bring to the boil, then reduce the heat and simmer for 5 minutes. Remove from the heat, sprinkle over ¼ teaspoon of xanthan gum to thicken, and stir well. If you prefer your soup a little thicker, add more, a tiny amount at a time, until the soup has reached your preferred consistency.

Crack the egg into a bowl and lightly beat with a fork.

Return the pan to the heat, then slowly drizzle the egg into the hot soup, while stirring. The egg will cook as it hits the hot soup and will become fine threads. Ladle into four warmed bowls and serve.

HOW *to* BATCH

Cool within 2 hours of cooking, then divide the cooked recipe into individual servings and freeze immediately. Allow to defrost then reheat, or reheat straight from frozen in the microwave or over a medium heat, stirring occasionally. Find detailed guidelines on reheating on page 11.

OVEN-BAKED RISOTTO *with* SMOKED SALMON *and* PEAS

🕐 **5 MINS** | 🍲 **30 MINS** | ✕ **SERVES 4**

Stove-cooked risotto requires concentration and can be time-consuming due to all the stirring and gradual adding of stock. We've created a nifty little oven-baked version that cuts out all the standing and stirring repeatedly. Sling it in the oven and let it bake away until ready. So much better!

→ use GF stock cubes

PER SERVING:
366 KCAL
65G CARBS

low-calorie cooking spray
½ medium onion, peeled and finely diced
300g risotto rice
2 tsp white wine vinegar
1 litre vegetable or chicken stock (2 vegetable or chicken stock cubes dissolved in 1 litre boiling water)
150g frozen peas
4 spring onions, trimmed and thinly sliced
100g smoked salmon, sliced
juice of 1 lemon
sea salt and freshly ground black pepper

Preheat the oven to 180°C (fan 160°C/gas mark 4).

Spray a casserole dish suitable for both hob and oven with low-calorie cooking spray. Add the finely diced onion and sauté over a medium–low heat for 3–4 minutes, until soft and translucent.

Add the rice to the pan, stir and sauté for another minute. Pour in the white wine vinegar and stock, stir and increase the heat. Bring to the boil, then cover with a tight-fitting lid and place in the oven.

After 20 minutes, remove from the oven and stir in the peas, spring onions, smoked salmon and lemon juice. Return to the oven for 5 more minutes. When cooked, season with salt and pepper and serve.

HOW *to* BATCH

Cool within 1 hour of cooking, then divide into individual portions and freeze immediately. Find detailed guidelines on storing and reheating rice on page 11.

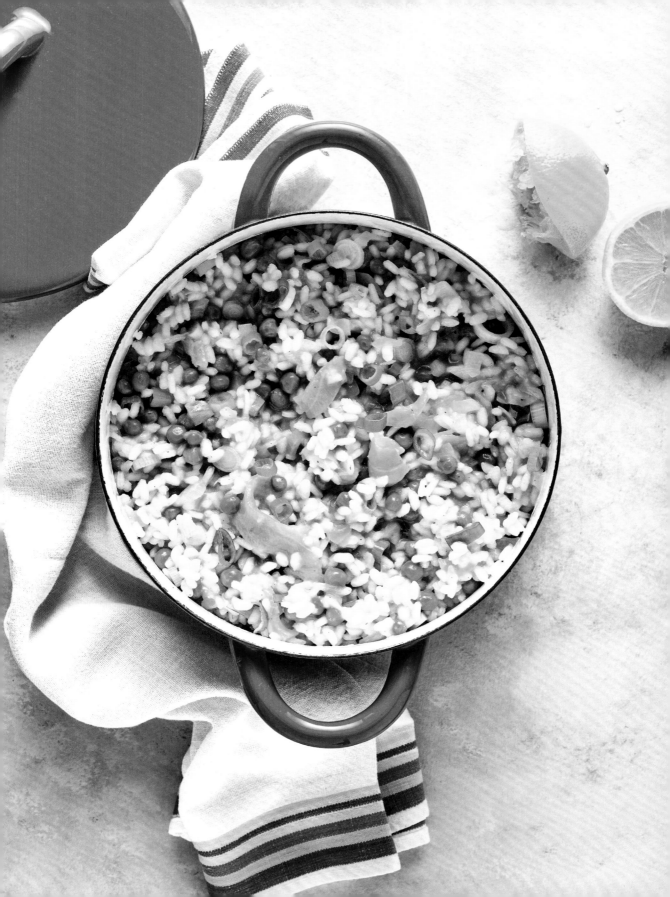

BUTTER BEAN *and* SWEET POTATO TIKKA MASALA

🕐 **10 MINS** | 🍲 **30 MINS** | ✕ **SERVES 4**

Butter beans are underrated, or so we say! Meaty, creamy and substantial, this filling bean is great to add to vegetarian dishes to bulk them up. The tikka masala sauce is very versatile and can be used with whatever you have in the cupboard, to make a quick and easy curry any day of the week.

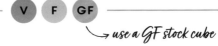

→ *use a GF stock cube*

PER SERVING:
232 KCAL
43G CARBS

low-calorie cooking spray
1 large onion, peeled and
    roughly chopped
1 red chilli, deseeded and chopped
3 garlic cloves, peeled and
    minced or grated
1cm (½in) piece of root ginger,
    peeled and grated
2 tbsp tomato puree
juice of ½ lemon
3 medium sweet potatoes,
    peeled and diced (about 425g)
250ml vegetable stock
    (1 vegetable stock cube
    dissolved in 250ml boiling water)
1 x 400g tin chopped tomatoes
sea salt and freshly ground
    black pepper
1 x 400g tin butter beans
75g spinach
10g fresh coriander, chopped
2 tbsp fat-free, natural yoghurt

FOR THE SPICE MIX
1 tsp paprika
1 tsp garam masala
1 tsp ground cumin
1 tsp ground coriander
¼ tsp ground cinnamon

Mix the spices together and set aside.

Spray a large frying pan or wok with low-calorie cooking spray. Add the chopped onion and chilli and cook over a medium heat for 4–5 minutes until the onions are soft and starting to colour. Add the garlic, ginger and spice mix, and continue cooking for another minute, allowing the spices to release their flavour, then add the tomato puree and lemon juice.

Using a food processor or stick blender, blitz the onion mix to a smooth paste, return to the pan (if using a food processor), add the sweet potato and stir until well coated. Add the stock and chopped tomatoes and season with salt and pepper. Stir and bring to the boil, then reduce the heat to low and simmer for 20 minutes, until the sweet potato is just cooked.

Drain the butter beans and add to the pan along with the spinach, then stir for 2–3 minutes, until the beans have heated through and the spinach has wilted.

Add the chopped coriander and stir through the yoghurt. Serve with your choice of accompaniments.

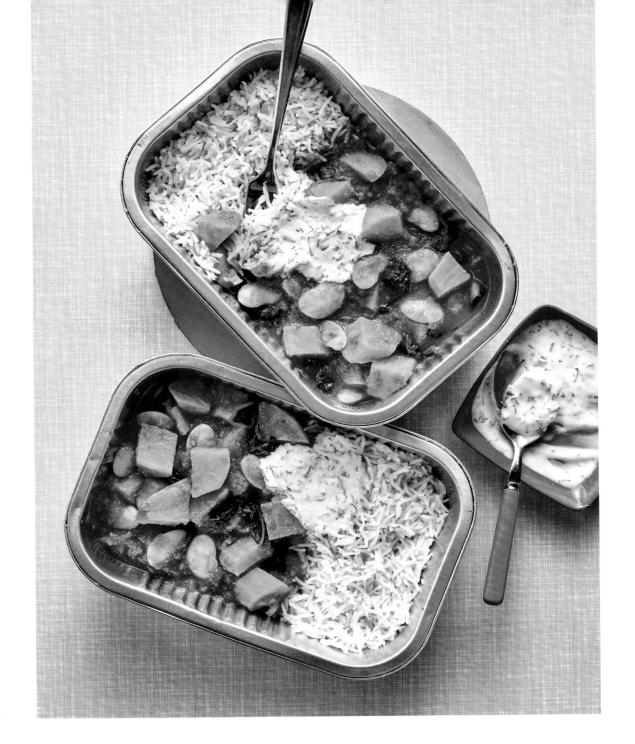

TO ACCOMPANY *(optional)*

50g uncooked rice per portion, cooked according to packet instructions (+ 173 kcal per 125g cooked serving)

HOW *to* BATCH

Cool within 1 hour of cooking, then divide into individual portions and freeze immediately. Find detailed guidelines on storing and reheating rice on page 11.

JAMBALAYA

🕐 **10 MINS** | 🍲 **30 MINS** | ✕ **SERVES 4**

Jambalaya, a traditional Louisiana dish, contains sausage as a staple ingredient. Its tomato-based sauce tastes incredible combined with the Cajun spice mix. You can add any meat you like to the recipe; we've chosen chicken to keep this meal everyday light, but you could use pork, prawns or both for an occasional indulgent twist.

F

PER SERVING:
398 KCAL
55.8G CARBS

low-calorie cooking spray
300g diced chicken
2 bell peppers, deseeded and diced
1 onion, peeled and finely diced
2 celery sticks, sliced
2 garlic cloves, peeled and minced or finely chopped
1–2 tbsp Cajun seasoning
1 tsp smoked paprika
½ tsp dried oregano
200g American long-grain rice
1 x 400g tin chopped tomatoes
400ml chicken stock (2 chicken stock cubes dissolved in 400ml boiling water)
1 tbsp Worcestershire sauce or Henderson's relish
3 cooked low-fat sausages, sliced

Spray a large, shallow casserole dish with low-calorie cooking spray, add the chicken and cook over a medium–high heat for 2–3 minutes. Add the peppers, onion and celery and cook for another minute.

Add the garlic, Cajun spice (according to taste), paprika and oregano, and cook for a further minute, to release the flavours.

Add the rice, chopped tomatoes, stock and Worcestershire sauce. Stir in the sausages and bring to the boil. Reduce the heat to low, cover and cook for 25 minutes, or until all the liquid has been absorbed and the rice is tender.

Tip

We've listed the sausages as pre-cooked as they are easier to slice if they've been left to cool down, but you could cook them according packet instructions as a first step.

HOW *to* BATCH

Cool within 1 hour of cooking, then divide into individual portions and freeze immediately. Find detailed guidelines on storing and reheating rice on page 11.

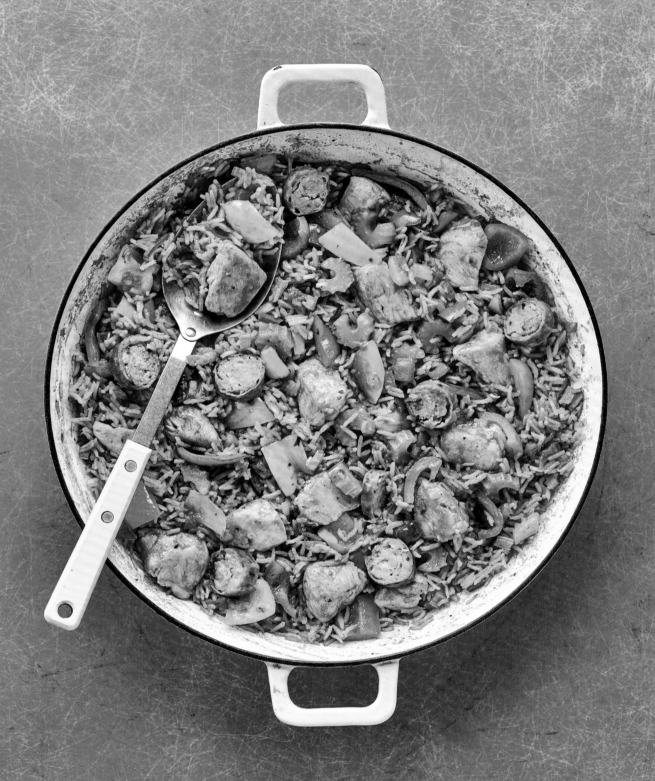

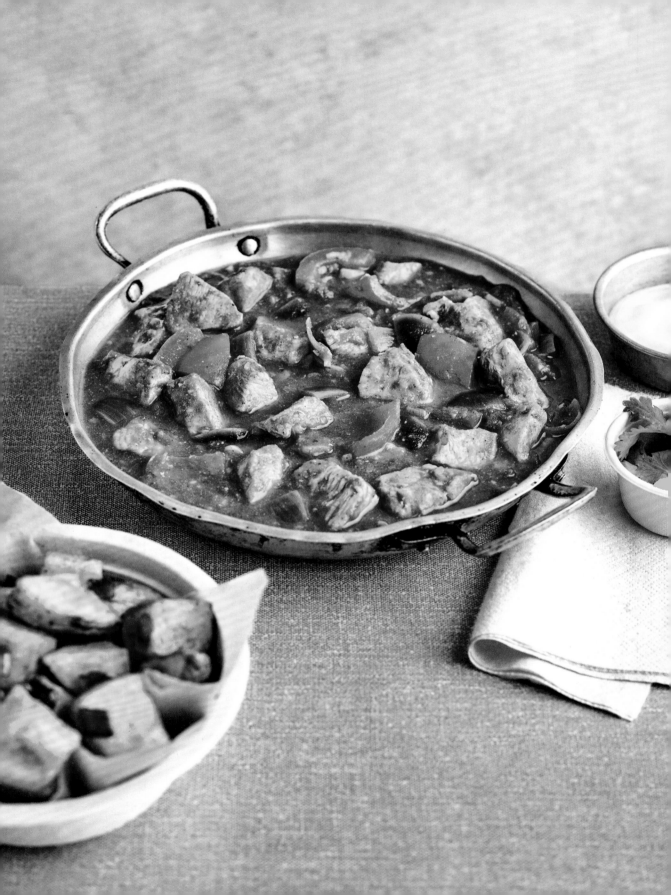

CHICKEN DOPIAZA *with* CUMIN ROAST POTATOES

🕐 **15 MINS** | 🍲 **30 MINS** | ✕ **SERVES 4**

This dopiaza is a South Asian dish. By cooking the recipe from scratch, you can eliminate the high oil content of a takeaway version, leaving you with the same amazingly spiced, onion-based dish, without the high calorie count.

F **GF**

→ use a GF stock cube

PER SERVING:
391 KCAL
65G CARBS

low-calorie cooking spray
2 red onions, peeled and diced
4 garlic cloves, peeled and finely chopped or grated
2.5cm (1in) piece of root ginger, peeled and grated
1 red chilli, deseeded and finely chopped
500g chicken breast (skin and visible fat removed), diced
1 tbsp garam masala
1 tsp ground cumin
1 tsp ground coriander
1 x 400g tin chopped tomatoes
200ml chicken stock (1 chicken stock cube dissolved in 200ml boiling water)
1 red pepper, deseeded and diced
1 tbsp chopped fresh coriander

FOR THE POTATOES
700g potatoes, scrubbed and cut into large dice (no need to peel)
½ red onion, peeled and finely diced
low-calorie cooking spray
sea salt and freshly ground black pepper
1½ tsp ground cumin

Preheat the oven to 190°C (fan 170°C/gas mark 5).

Parboil the potatoes for 5 minutes. Drain and place in a bowl. Add the diced red onion, spray with some low-calorie cooking spray, season with salt and pepper, sprinkle the ground cumin over and mix well. Tip onto an oven tray and cook for 30 minutes or until the potatoes are cooked through and golden brown.

Next, prepare the curry. Spray a large heavy-based frying pan or wok with some low-calorie cooking spray, then add the diced onions, garlic, ginger and chilli and cook over a medium heat for 5 minutes.

Add the chicken to the pan and cook for another 5 minutes until the meat starts to brown slightly. Stir in the garam masala, cumin and coriander and continue to cook for another minute. Add the chopped tomatoes and stock, stir well, then bring it back to the boil. Turn the heat down and simmer for 15 minutes.

Add the red pepper and allow to cook for another 3 minutes. Stir in the coriander and serve with the cumin roast potatoes, or whatever you fancy.

HOW *to* BATCH

Cool within 2 hours of cooking, then divide the cooked recipe into individual servings (minus the potato accompaniment) and freeze immediately. Find detailed guidelines on reheating on page 11.

MEDITERRANEAN TUNA PASTA

🕐 **15 MINS** | 🍲 **40 MINS** | ✗ **SERVES 6**

A firm family favourite, this tomatoey pasta dish is packed with veggies and topped with both Cheddar and feta cheese for a super-cheesy yet traditionally Mediterranean flavour. It also works very well with chicken. At only 398 calories a portion, you won't believe how filling and delicious slimming food can be!

— F —

PER SERVING:
398 KCAL
55.8G CARBS

low-calorie cooking spray
4 red onions, peeled and
    finely chopped
2 carrots, peeled and finely
    chopped (200g)
1 celery stick, finely chopped
6 garlic cloves, peeled and minced
250ml vegetable stock
    (2 vegetable stock cubes
    dissolved in 250ml boiling water)
2 courgettes
2 red peppers
2 x 120g tins tuna (in water or
    brine), drained
1 x 250g carton passata
2 x 400g tins chopped tomatoes
2 tbsp balsamic vinegar
1 tbsp Worcestershire sauce or
    Henderson's relish
1 tbsp dried oregano
1 tbsp dried basil
1 tbsp sweet paprika
sea salt and freshly ground
    black pepper
300g dried pasta
80g reduced-fat Cheddar
65g reduced-fat feta cheese
dried paprika flakes and fresh
    basil, to serve (optional)

Preheat the oven to 200°C (fan 180°C/gas mark 6).

Spray a large saucepan with some low-calorie cooking spray, add the onions, carrots, celery and minced garlic and sauté for a few minutes over a medium heat until softened. Add the stock and simmer for another 5 minutes.

Quarter and slice the courgettes, then deseed and thinly slice the red peppers. Add the courgettes, peppers, drained tuna, passata and tinned tomatoes to the saucepan. Add the balsamic vinegar, Worcestershire sauce, oregano, basil, paprika, and some salt and pepper to the pan and stir. Add the lid to the pan and leave to simmer while you cook the pasta (about 6 minutes).

Cook the pasta in a separate pan of boiling salted water according to the packet instructions, but for half the time. (If the cooking time is 12 minutes, cook for 6.) Once the pasta is part cooked, drain and add to a roasting dish. Pour over the contents of the saucepan and mix together.

Grate the Cheddar and crumble the feta. Sprinkle over the top of the pasta bake. Put the roasting dish in the oven for 20 minutes.

When ready, take out of the oven and sprinkle over the fresh basil and the paprika flakes (if using) and serve.

HOW *to* BATCH

Cool within 2 hours of cooking, then divide the cooked recipe into individual servings and freeze immediately. Find detailed guidelines on reheating on page 11.

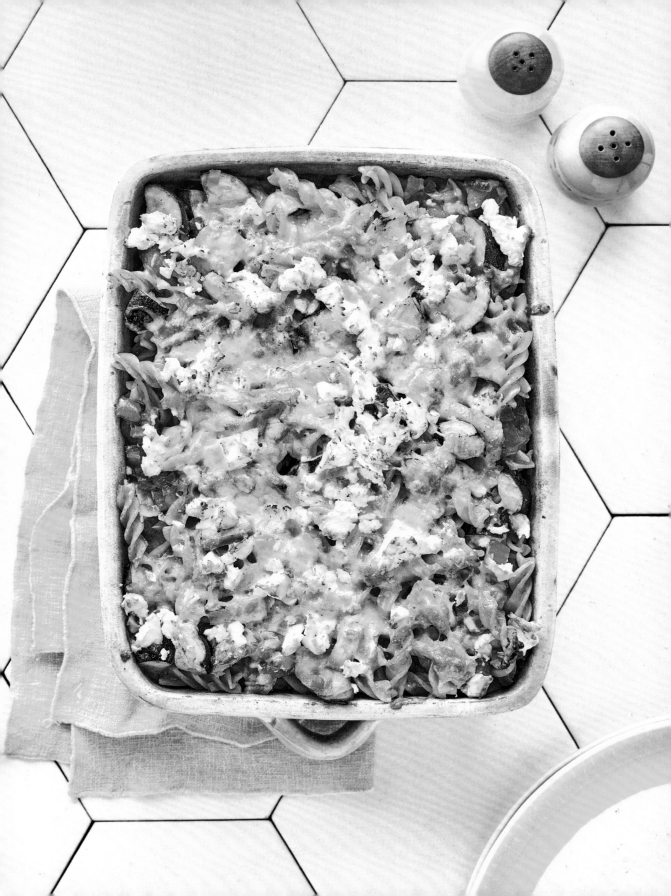

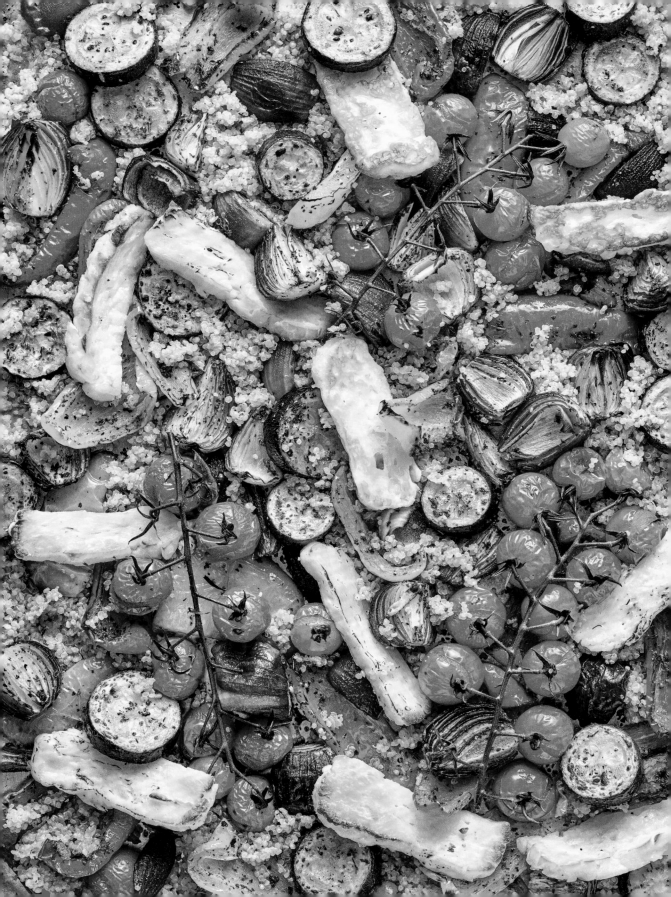

ROASTED VEGETABLE *and* HALLOUMI QUINOA

🕐 **5 MINS** | 🍲 **50 MINS** | ✕ **SERVES 6**

Quinoa is a grain that looks a bit like couscous but is higher in protein, which keeps you feeling full for longer. It makes the perfect base for these tasty roasted vegetables, but you can also swap for pasta, couscous or another grain if you wish. Melted halloumi takes it to the next level!

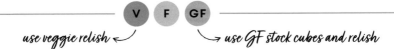

V F GF

use veggie relish ←   → *use GF stock cubes and relish*

PER SERVING:
373 KCAL
51G CARBS

2 large red onions, peeled and quartered

2 courgettes, sliced into 1cm (½ in)-thick discs

4 peppers (mixture of red and yellow), deseeded and each cut into 8 pieces

350g cherry tomatoes, left whole

2 tbsp balsamic vinegar

1 tbsp Worcestershire sauce or Henderson's relish

low-calorie cooking spray

2 tsp dried oregano

2 tsp dried basil

1 tbsp garlic granules

300g dried quinoa

2 vegetable stock cubes, crumbled

1 tsp lemon juice

135g reduced-fat halloumi, thinly sliced

sea salt and freshly ground black pepper

Preheat the oven to 220°C (fan 200°C/gas mark 7).

Add all the vegetables to a large roasting dish. Drizzle the balsamic vinegar and Worcestershire sauce over them. Coat them with low-calorie cooking spray and sprinkle the oregano, basil and garlic granules on top.

Place the roasting dish in the middle of the hot oven for 25 minutes. Turn the vegetables, spray with more low-calorie cooking spray and cook for another 20 minutes. When it's ready the vegetables should be cooked through but still hold their shape, deeper in colour and crispy at the edges but not burnt.

Meanwhile, cook the quinoa according to the packet instructions. Though it looks similar to couscous, quinoa needs takes longer to cook on the hob. Add the stock cubes to the quinoa when you add the water to cook it. When the quinoa is cooked, fluff it up with a fork and stir in the lemon juice.

When the roasted vegetables are done, take the tray out of the oven and mix the quinoa into it. Season with salt and pepper to taste. Lay the halloumi slices on the top of the vegetable-quinoa mix and place the tray back into the oven for 5 minutes, until the halloumi has melted. Remove from the oven and serve.

HOW *to* BATCH

Cool within 2 hours of cooking, then divide the cooked recipe into individual servings (with or without the halloumi) and freeze immediately. Find detailed guidelines on reheating on page 11.

BEEF KOFTA CURRY

🕐 **10 MINS** | 🍲 **35 MINS** | ✕ **SERVES 4**

Everyone loves a good curry. Cooking one from scratch means you can still indulge in a Friday-night curry without having to worry about the indulgence. This recipe, using lean minced beef made into meatballs, takes the same amount of time as it would to wait for your curry house to deliver, and tastes absolutely amazing. The perfect Fakeaway.

F **GF**

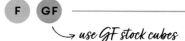

→ *use GF stock cubes*

PER SERVING:
201 KCAL
12G CARBS

low-calorie cooking spray
1 onion, peeled and diced
3 garlic cloves, peeled and
    crushed or grated
1 tbsp curry powder
1 tbsp tomato puree
750ml beef stock (2 beef
    stock cubes dissolved in
    750ml boiling water)
225g butternut squash, peeled
    and chopped
400g 5%-fat minced beef
10g fresh coriander, chopped
sea salt and freshly ground
    black pepper
75g fat-free natural yoghurt

TO ACCOMPANY *(optional)*
50g uncooked rice per portion,
    cooked according to packet
    instructions (+ 173 kcal per 125g
    cooked serving)

Spray a saucepan with low-calorie cooking spray, add the diced onion and cook over a medium heat for 4–5 minutes until it is soft and beginning to brown. Add two-thirds of the garlic and the curry powder and continue cooking for 1 minute, allowing the flavour of the spices to be released. Add the tomato puree, stir well, then add the stock. Add the butternut squash, stir and bring to the boil. Reduce the heat and simmer for 20–25 minutes.

Meanwhile, make the meatballs. Place the minced beef in a bowl with the remaining garlic and half the chopped coriander and season with salt and pepper. Mix well, then divide into twelve even pieces and roll into balls.

Spray a wok or a frying pan with low-calorie cooking spray. Add the meatballs to the pan and fry over a medium–high heat, turning frequently, for 5–10 minutes, until the meatballs are browned on all sides and cooked through. Place to one side.

When the butternut squash is soft, remove from the heat and blitz the mixture with a stick blender until smooth.

Pour the sauce into the pan with the meatballs, stir well, cover and simmer for 5 minutes. Remove from the heat, stir in the yoghurt and the remaining coriander, and serve.

HOW *to* BATCH

Cool within 2 hours of cooking, then divide the cooked recipe into individual servings (roughly three kofta per portion) and freeze immediately. Find detailed guidelines on reheating on page 11.

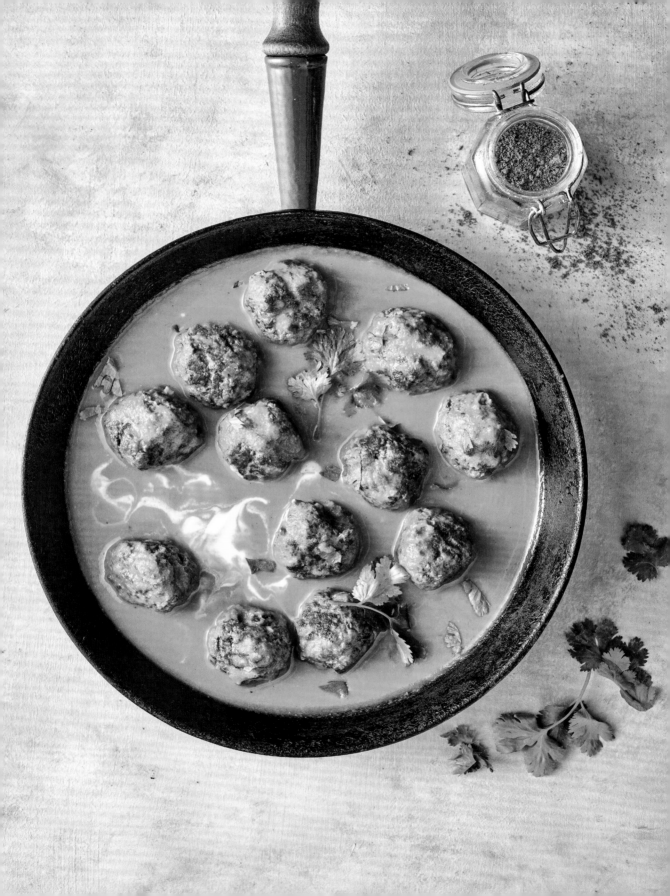

PASTA ARRABBIATA

🕐 **5 MINS** | 🍲 **15 MINS** | ✕ **SERVES 4**

'Arrabbiata' means 'angry' in Italian, and this pasta dish has this name due to the spicy dried chilli in it. Our version of this classic Italian dish has a rich tomato sauce, with herbs and the all-important red chilli flakes. You can adapt the heat to suit your taste – use a little more or less depending on how 'angry' you like it!

PER SERVING:
356 KCAL
65G CARBS

1 red pepper, deseeded
low-calorie cooking spray
4 garlic cloves, peeled and
    chopped
1 tsp dried chilli flakes
1 x 400g tin chopped tomatoes
2 tbsp tomato puree
1 tsp dried oregano
1 tsp dried basil
sea salt and freshly ground
    black pepper
320g pasta
fresh basil leaves, torn, to serve

Dice the red pepper into 1cm (½in) square pieces. Spray a large frying pan with low-calorie cooking spray. Place on a low heat, crush the garlic cloves into the frying pan, add the chilli flakes and red pepper and cook for a couple of minutes until the pepper starts to soften.

Add the tinned tomatoes, tomato puree and dried herbs. Mix well, season with salt and pepper to taste, and turn the heat up to medium–high. Stir frequently for around 10 minutes as the sauce reduces and you cook the pasta.

While the sauce is cooking, bring a large saucepan of salted water to the boil and cook the pasta according to the packet instructions.

Once the pasta has cooked, drain and add to the sauce.

Combine the pasta and sauce, ensuring all of the pasta is well coated. Serve with a sprinkle of fresh basil.

HOW *to* BATCH

Cool the sauce within 2 hours of cooking, then divide it into individual servings and freeze immediately. Find detailed guidelines on reheating on page 11.

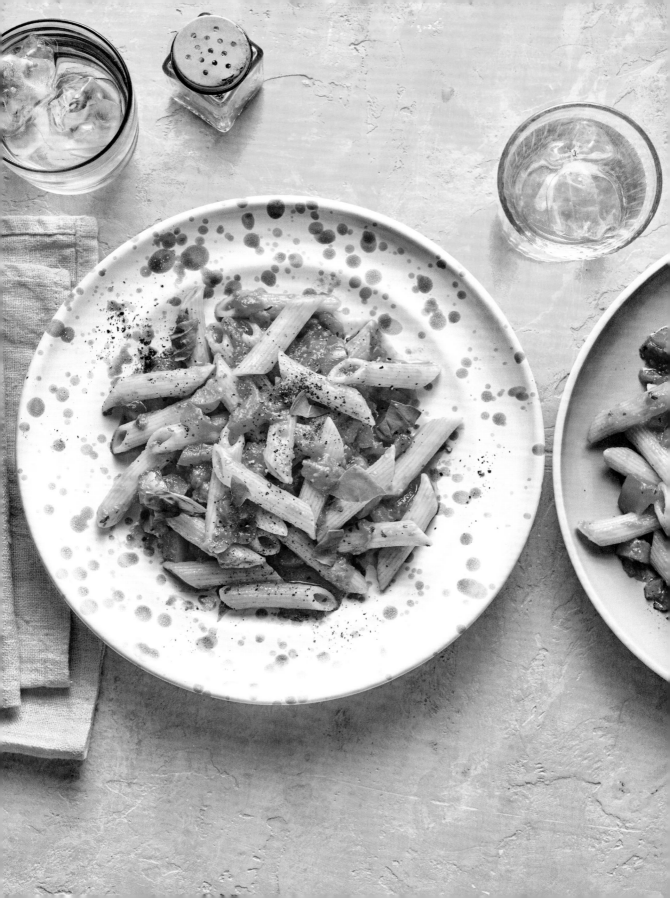

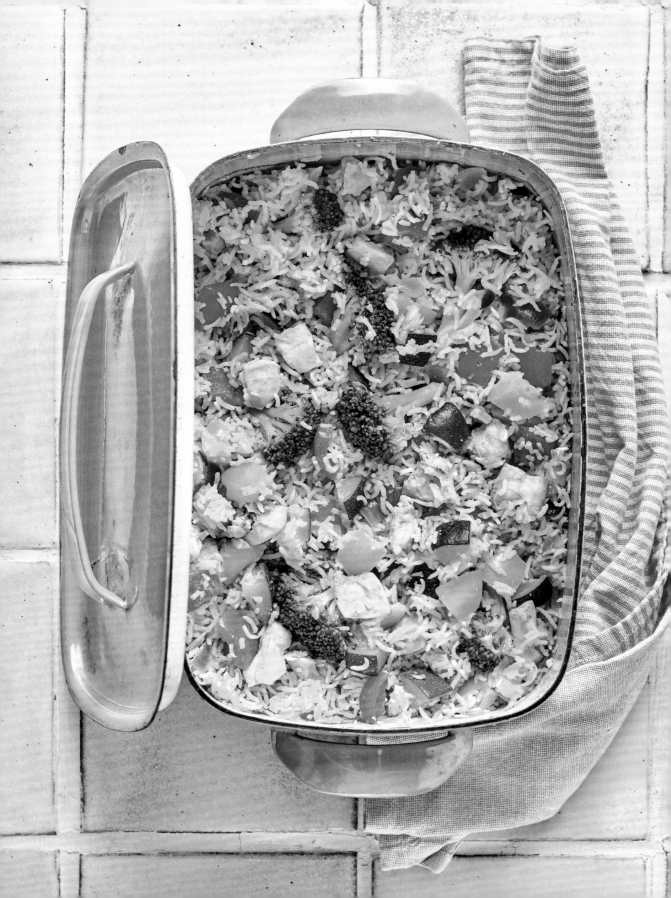

CHICKEN, VEGETABLE *and* RICE BAKE

🕐 **5 MINS** | 🍲 **50 MINS** | ✗ **SERVES 6**

This simple bake is fuss-free and really easy to make. We've chosen an array of vegetables for this dish and the beauty of it is that you can choose whatever you like; tomatoes, cauliflower, carrots – anything goes! The curry powder and turmeric add colour and a mild savoury flavour to the rice.

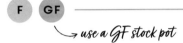

F **GF**

↳ *use a GF stock pot*

PER SERVING:
374 KCAL
43G CARBS

600g chicken thigh fillets (skin and visible fat removed) cut into 2cm (¾ in) pieces
300g basmati rice
600ml chicken stock (1 chicken stock pot dissolved in 600ml boiling water)
150g broccoli, cut into small florets
1 yellow pepper, deseeded and cut into 2cm (¾ in) dice
1 red pepper, deseeded and cut into 2cm (¾ in) dice
1 small onion, peeled and roughly chopped
1 courgette, cut into 2cm (¾ in) dice
1 tsp mild curry powder
1 tsp ground turmeric
1 tsp garlic granules
sea salt and freshly ground black pepper

Preheat the oven to 170°C (fan 150°C/gas mark 3).

Place all of the ingredients in a large, ovenproof baking dish. Mix well, season with salt and pepper and place in the oven for 25 minutes.

Remove from the oven, stir and put back into the oven for another 20–25 minutes, until the rice is cooked through. Serve while piping hot.

HOW *to* BATCH

Cool within 1 hour of cooking, then divide into individual portions and freeze immediately. Find detailed guidelines on storing and reheating rice on page 11.

VEGGIE SPAGHETTI BOLOGNESE

⏱ **5 MINS** | 🍲 **30 MINS** | ✕ **SERVES 4**

Whether you are a vegetarian or just looking for a meat-free recipe, this Veggie Spaghetti Bolognese is perfect to make for the whole family. It's packed with wholesome vegetables and filling lentils, which bulk up the mix with goodness while tasting just as good! Serve with Parmesan if you don't mind the calories.

V F GF

→ use GF stock cubes and spaghetti

PER SERVING:
386 KCAL
74G CARBS

low-calorie cooking spray
1 onion, peeled and finely diced
3 garlic cloves, peeled and crushed
1 medium carrot, peeled and finely diced
1 small courgette, finely diced
1 x 400g tin green lentils, drained
100g mushrooms, sliced
3 tbsp tomato puree
1 x 400g tin chopped tomatoes
1 x 500g carton passata
1 tbsp dried oregano
1 tbsp dried basil
1 red wine stock pot
1 vegetable stock pot
sea salt and freshly ground black pepper
240g spaghetti

Spray a large frying pan with low-calorie cooking spray, place on a medium heat, add the onion, garlic, carrot and courgette and cook for 5 minutes until starting to soften. Add all of the other ingredients, stir, and simmer over a medium heat for 25 minutes, until the sauce has reduced slightly and the vegetables are soft.

While the Bolognese is cooking, cook the spaghetti according to the packet instructions. Serve as soon as the pasta is cooked.

HOW *to* BATCH

Cool within 2 hours of cooking, then divide the bolognese sauce into individual servings (minus the spaghetti accompaniment) and freeze immediately. Find detailed guidelines on reheating on page 11.

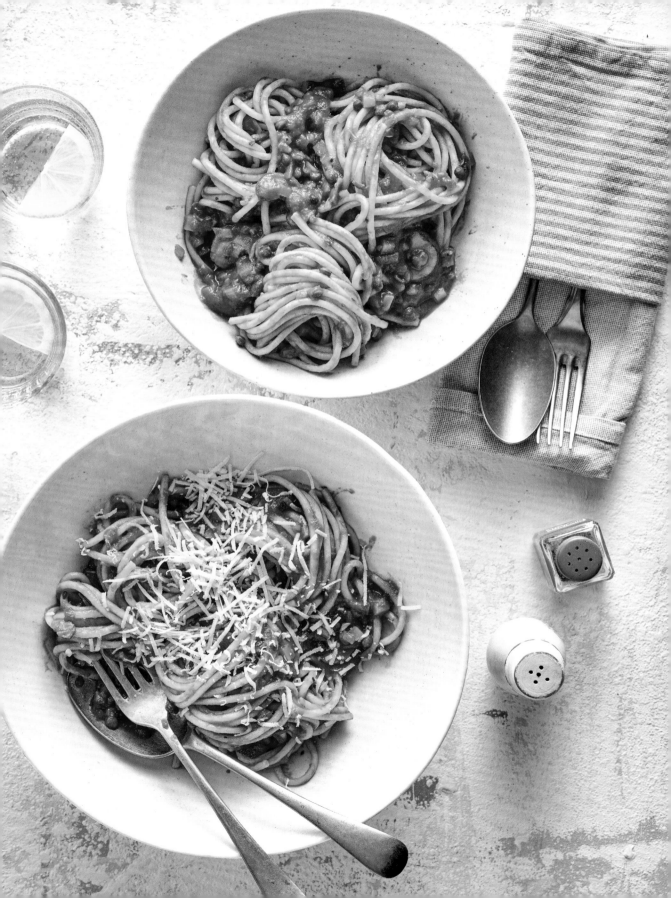

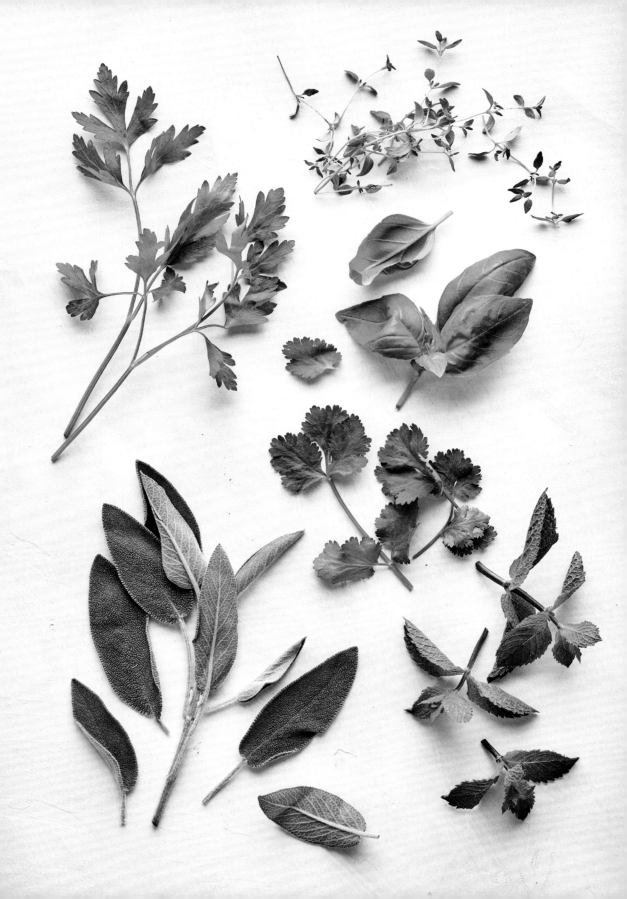

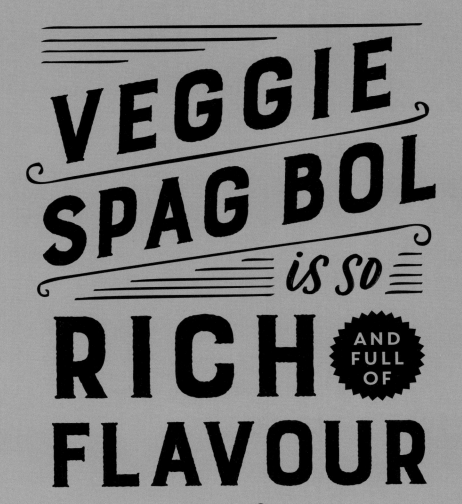

VEGGIE SPAG BOL *is so* RICH AND FULL OF FLAVOUR

CHARLENE

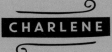

CHICKEN DOPIAZA is very *tasty* and incredibly simple to make.

CATHY

Made the **CHICKEN, VEGETABLE + RICE BAKE** tonight and what a *hit!*

JENNY

CABBAGE ROLLS

🕐 **10 MINS** | 🍲 **45 MINS** | ✗ **SERVES 6**

These cabbage rolls are packed with flavour. Found in many Eastern European countries, they're made in a similar way to an enchilada, but with an added cabbage component instead of the wrap, and a richer sauce – boosting your veg intake and reducing the calories for this calorie-light but substantial meal.

F **GF**

↳ *use a GF stock pot and relish*

PER SERVING:
359 KCAL
36G CARBS

1 large head of cabbage, whole
100g uncooked rice
2 large onions, peeled and
    finely chopped
low-calorie cooking spray
500g 5%-fat minced beef
2 tsp Worcestershire sauce
2 tsp garlic granules
1 tsp dried parsley
2 tbsp tomato puree
1 red wine or beef stock pot
sea salt and freshly ground
    black pepper

FOR THE SAUCE
1 x 400g tin chopped tomatoes
1 x 500g carton passata
1 tbsp white wine vinegar
1 tsp Worcestershire sauce
    or Henderson's relish
1 tsp granulated sweetener

TO ACCOMPANY *(optional)*
80g steamed veg
    (+ 38 kcal per serving)

Preheat the oven to 220°C (fan 200°C/gas mark 7).

Place the head of cabbage in a large saucepan and cover with water. Bring to the boil, reduce the heat, then simmer for 5 minutes with the lid on. Drain and leave to cool so that you can handle it.

In a separate saucepan cook the rice according to the packet instructions. While the cabbage and rice are cooking, spray a frying pan with some low-calorie cooking spray, add the onions and cook over a medium heat for 5 minutes until soft.

In a bowl mix the cooked onions, cooked rice, raw beef mince, Worcestershire sauce, garlic, parsley, tomato puree and stock pot and season with salt and pepper.

Cut the hard stem off the bottom of the cabbage. Carefully peel off the leaves. Take a small handful of the beef mix and place in the centre of a cabbage leaf. Fold in the sides, then roll up the leaf so that you have a small parcel. Lay seam side down in a roasting dish and repeat until the beef and rice mixture is used up.

Mix the sauce ingredients together, season with salt and pepper and pour the sauce over the cabbage rolls. Place in the middle of the oven for 30 minutes. Remove from the oven and serve.

HOW *to* BATCH

Cool within 1 hour of cooking, then divide into individual portions and freeze immediately. Find detailed guidelines on storing and reheating rice on page 11. You can also finely chop and freeze leftover raw cabbage and add it to stews and soups.

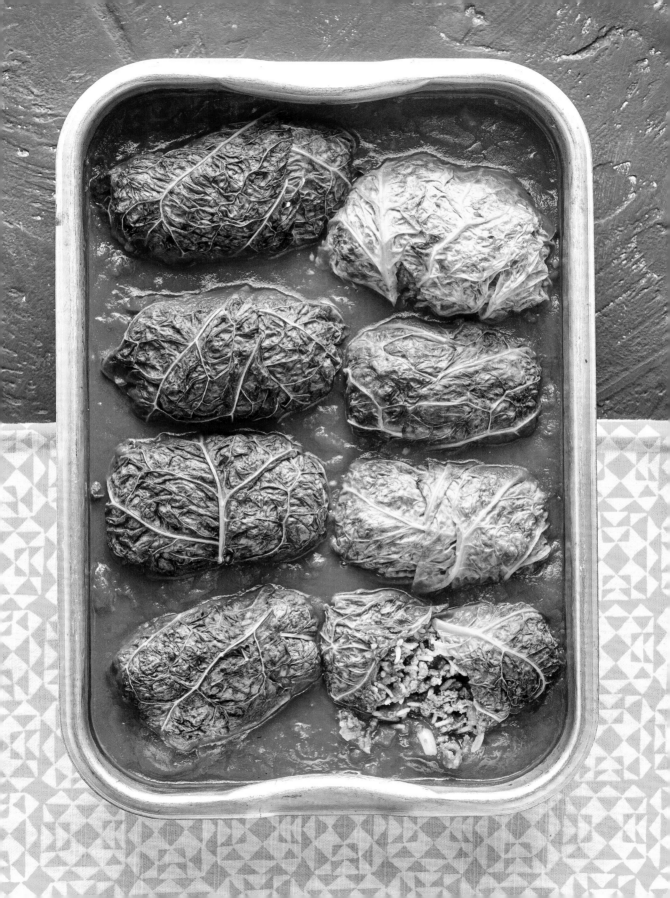

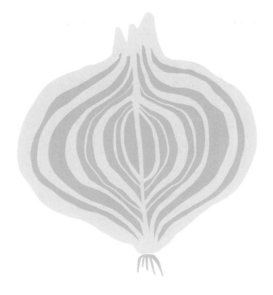

STEWS and SOUPS

SOPA CRIOLLA

🕐 **10 MINS** | 🍲 **30 MINS** | ✕ **SERVES 4**

This warming soup originates from Peru and is traditionally served with a fried egg on top. The soup has a smoky, tomato flavour and the pasta adds some bulk and filling power. It takes no time at all to prepare and is perfect served on a chilly winter evening.

F

PER SERVING:
313 KCAL
28G CARBS

60g wholemeal bread
low-calorie cooking spray
sea salt and freshly ground
   black pepper
1 onion, peeled and diced
200g lean, quick-cooking beef
   steak (such as medallions or
   rump), thinly sliced
½ tsp dried chipotle flakes
½ tsp smoked paprika
1 garlic clove, peeled and minced
½ tsp dried oregano
2 tomatoes, diced
2 tbsp tomato puree
1 litre beef stock (2 beef stock
   cubes dissolved in 1 litre
   boiling water)
75g angel hair pasta (or spaghetti)
4 eggs

Preheat the oven to 200°C (fan 180°C/gas mark 6).

Cut the bread into 1cm (½in) cubes, place on a baking tray and spray with low-calorie cooking spray. Season with salt and pepper and place in the oven for 10 minutes, until crisp and golden. (If you are cooking the soup in advance, to freeze and have another day, leave out this stage and cook the croutons when you are ready to serve the soup.)

Sauté the onion and sliced steak in a large saucepan over a medium heat for 4 minutes, until the onion softens and starts to brown. Add the chipotle flakes, paprika, garlic and oregano, and stir well to coat. Next, add the tomatoes and tomato puree and cook for 1 minute. Pour in the stock, stir well, then turn up the heat and bring to a boil. Add the angel hair pasta or spaghetti, reduce the heat and simmer for 5 minutes, until the pasta is cooked. If using spaghetti, increase the cooking time to 10–12 minutes. (At this point, the soup can be frozen once cooled – defrost fully before reheating.)

Using low-calorie cooking spray, fry the eggs. Ladle the soup into four bowls, sprinkle on the croutons and place the fried eggs on top, before serving.

Tip

This is traditionally made using *aji panca,* a smoky Peruvian chilli pepper. We use chipotle flakes and paprika to recreate the taste, but if you find *aji panca* paste, use that!

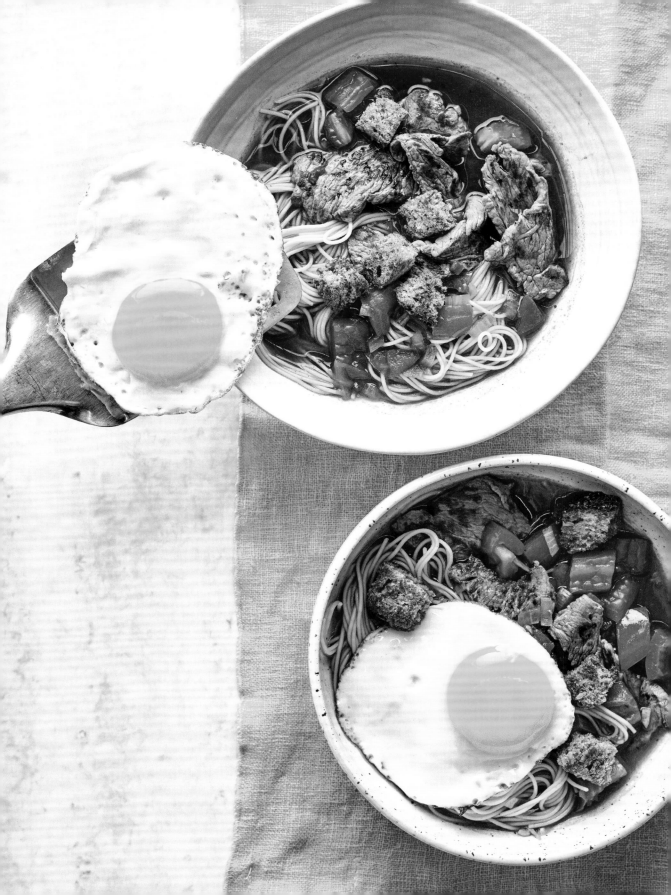

BEEF *and* SWEET POTATO STEW

🕐 **15 MINS** | 🍲 **VARIABLE** (SEE BELOW) | ✕ **SERVES 4**

If you ask us, on a cold, autumnal evening, there are few better things than walking through the door to the smell of a slow-cooked stew, ready and waiting for dinner. If only other parts of our lives could take care of themselves the same way! This is super easy to prep and can be cooked in the oven or slow cooker, making it the ideal midweek family meal.

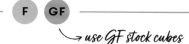

F GF

→ *use GF stock cubes*

PER SERVING:
345 KCAL
40G CARBS

low-calorie cooking spray
400g lean, diced stewing beef
1 large onion, peeled and diced
2 medium carrots, peeled
   and diced
1 celery stick, diced
½ tsp dried thyme
½ tsp garlic granules
1 tbsp tomato puree
1 x 400g tin chopped tomatoes
500ml beef stock (3 beef
   stock cubes dissolved in
   500ml boiling water)
2 tsp red wine vinegar
500g sweet potato, peeled
   and diced
sea salt and freshly ground
   black pepper
fresh thyme, to serve (optional)

OVEN METHOD
🍲 **2–2½ HRS**

Preheat the oven to 160°C (fan 140°C/gas mark 3).

Spray an ovenproof casserole dish with low-calorie cooking spray. Place over a medium–high heat, add the beef and fry for 4–5 minutes, until it is starting to brown. Add the onion, carrots, celery, thyme, garlic granules and tomato puree and stir well. Add the tomatoes, stock and red wine vinegar then stir in the sweet potato. Cover with a tight-fitting lid and place in the preheated oven.

Check after 2 hours. Gently squash some of the sweet potato and stir. This will thicken the gravy. Add a little water if the stew is drying out. When cooked, the meat should fall apart easily. Season with salt and pepper to taste and serve, garnished with fresh thyme, if using. The stew can be frozen once cooled – defrost thoroughly, and reheat until piping hot.

SLOW COOKER METHOD
🍲 **7 HRS**

Fry the beef as described in the method above.

Place all the other ingredients in the slow cooker. Add the meat and stir well. Cook on Low for 7 hours.

After 7 hours, gently squash some of the sweet potato and stir. This will thicken the gravy. Season with salt and pepper to taste and serve. The stew can be frozen once cooled.

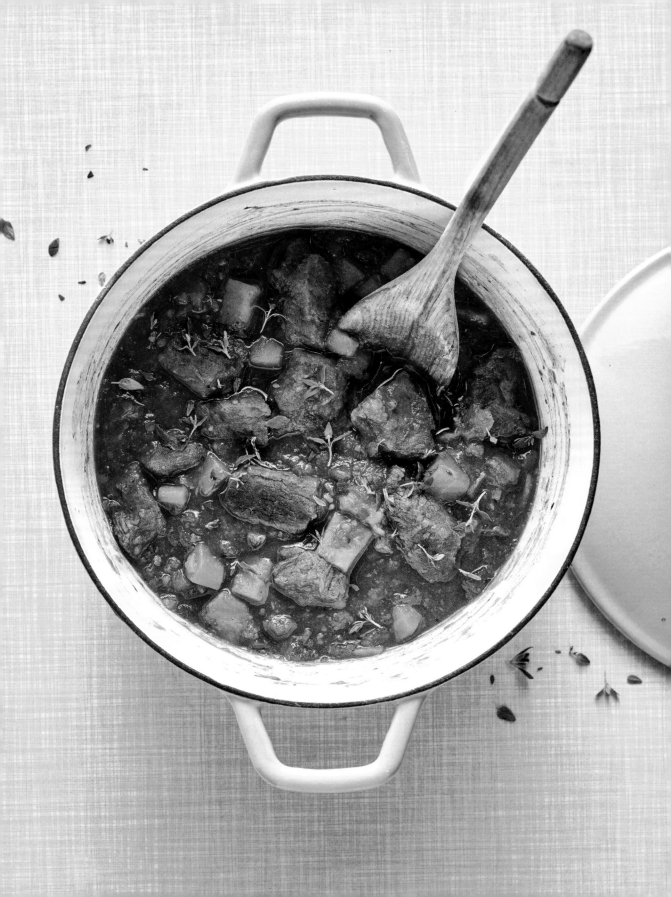

CHERRY COLA PULLED PORK

🕐 **15 MINS** | 🍲 **VARIABLE** (SEE BELOW) | 🍴 **SERVES 6**

Pulled pork is a great dish, and this version uses low-calorie soda to give it some smoky sweetness. Don't worry if you're not usually a fan of this pop, the final result is a tasty BBQ sauce and you'd never guess how it was made!

F **GF**

↳ *use GF stock cube and relish*

PER SERVING:
356 KCAL
15G CARBS

1.5kg pork shoulder joint
(weight including fat)
4 white onions, peeled and
roughly sliced
660ml diet cherry cola (we also
like Dr Pepper)
2 tsp Worcestershire sauce
or Henderson's relish
1 pork stock cube, crumbled
1 tsp smoked paprika
1 tbsp garlic granules
1 tsp onion granules
sea salt and freshly ground
black pepper
4 tbsp tomato puree
1 tbsp balsamic vinegar

TO ACCOMPANY *(optional)*
80g steamed veg
(+ 38 kcal per serving)

Tip
If you have a lot of sauce left over, save it in the fridge or freeze it. You can use it as a BBQ sauce with other dishes.

OVEN METHOD
🍲 **2 HRS 35 MINS**

Preheat the oven to 170°C (150°C/gas mark 3).

Remove the visible fat from the pork shoulder joint, cut the meat into large chunks about the size of a matchbox then put it in a large ovenproof casserole dish. Add the pork, onions, cherry cola, Worcestershire sauce, stock cube, paprika, garlic granules, onion granules and a pinch each of salt and pepper. Stir to combine.

Put the lid on the dish and place in the middle of the hot oven for 2½ hours. Once the meat is ready it will be tender and falling apart when you push your fork into it. Depending on how lean the meat is, there may be some fat that has risen to the top of the stock. Skim the fat off with a spoon and discard. Remove the meat and place in a separate bowl.

If your casserole dish can be used on the hob, remove from the oven and place over a medium heat. If it can't, transfer the onions and stock into a saucepan. Stir in the tomato puree and balsamic vinegar and simmer the onions and remaining stock for 5 minutes, or until the stock has reduced by half. Use a stick blender to blend the onions and stock. You should be left with a thick BBQ sauce. If it's still too thin, reduce further over a medium heat.

While the sauce is reducing, shred the pork using two forks. Pour the sauce over the pork – just enough to coat the pork well. Serve hot. The dish can also be frozen once cooled – defrost fully then reheat until piping hot.

More methods overleaf...

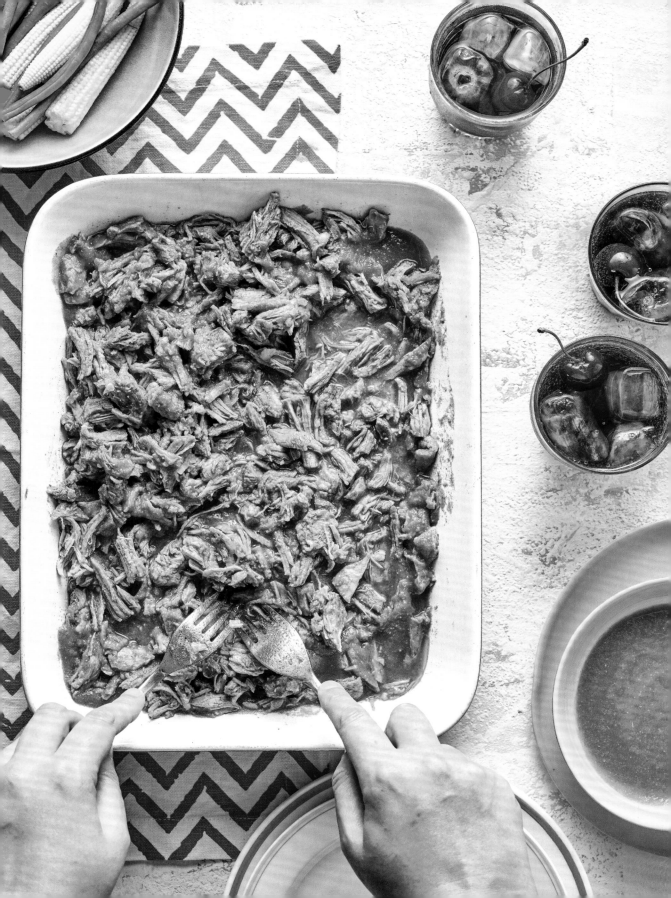

PRESSURE COOKER METHOD
🍲 35 MINS

Remove the visible fat from the pork shoulder joint and cut the meat into large chunks about the size of a matchbox. Add the pork, onions, cherry cola, Worcestershire sauce, stock cube, paprika, garlic granules, onion granules and salt and pepper to the pressure cooker. Stir to combine.

Place the lid on and pressure cook for 30 minutes. You can use Natural Pressure Release (NPR) or quick release. Once the meat is ready it will be tender and falling apart when you push your fork into it. Depending on how lean the meat is there may be some fat that has risen to the top of the stock. Skim the fat off with a spoon and discard. Remove the meat and place in a separate bowl.

Set the pressure cooker to Sauté. Stir in the tomato puree and balsamic vinegar and simmer the onions and remaining stock for 5 minutes, or until the stock has reduced by half. Use a stick blender to blend the onions and stock. You should be left with a thick BBQ sauce. If it's still too thin, reduce further on the Sauté setting.

While the sauce is reducing, shred the pork using two forks. Pour the sauce over the pork – just enough to coat the pork well. Serve hot. The dish can also be frozen once cooled.

SLOW COOKER METHOD
🍲 5–10 HRS

Remove the visible fat from the pork shoulder joint and cut the meat into large chunks about the size of a matchbox. Add the pork, onions, cherry cola, Worcestershire sauce, stock cube, paprika, garlic granules, onion granules and salt and pepper to the slow cooker. Stir to combine.

Place the lid on and cook on High for 5 hours or on Low for 10 hours. Once the meat is ready it will be tender and falling apart when you push your fork into it. Depending on how lean the meat was there may be some fat that has risen to the top of the stock. Skim the fat off with a spoon and discard. Remove the meat and place in a separate bowl.

Pour the liquid and onions into a saucepan. Over a medium heat stir in the tomato puree and balsamic vinegar and simmer the onions and remaining stock for 5 minutes, or until the stock has reduced by half. Use a stick blender to blend the onions and stock. You should be left with a thick BBQ sauce. If it's still too thin, reduce further over a medium heat.

While the sauce is reducing, shred the pork using two forks. Pour the sauce over the pork – just enough to coat the pork well. Serve hot. The dish can also be frozen once cooled.

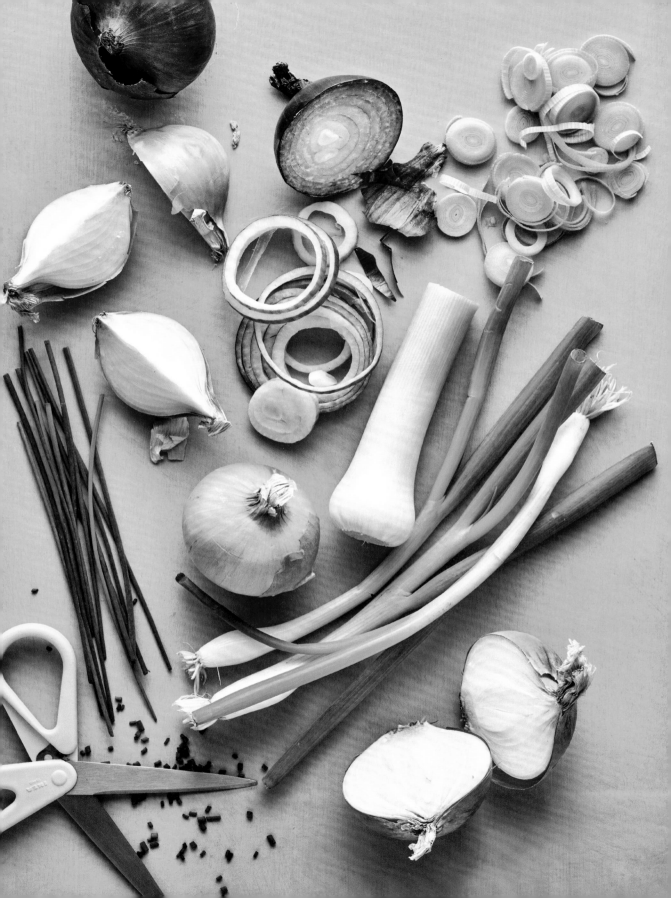

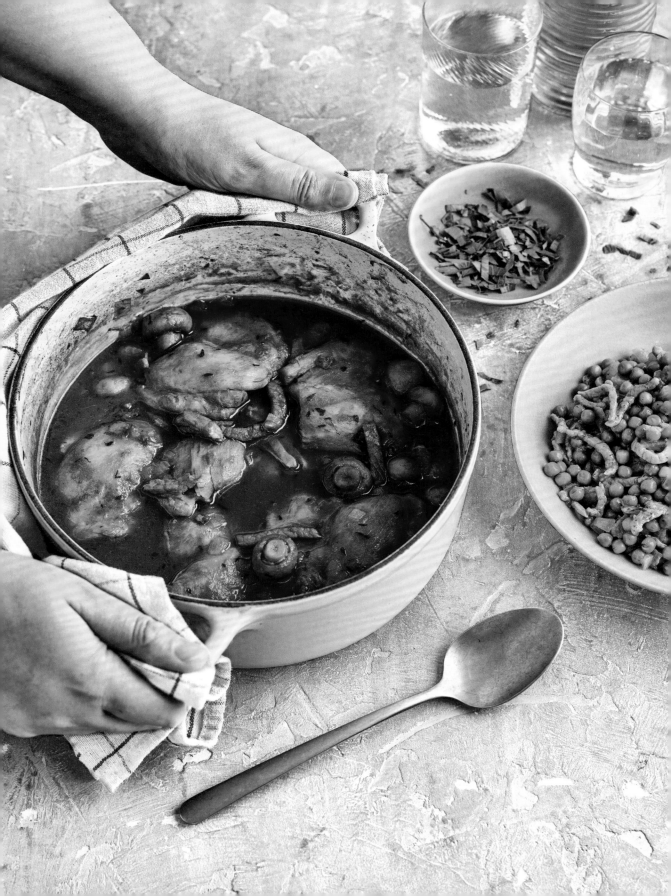

COQ *au* VIN

🕐 **10 MINS** | 🍲 **1 HR 40 MINS** | ✕ **SERVES 4**

How do we make wine low calorie? I regret to inform you that we're not reverse Jesus, turning wine back into water! The fairly recent invention of the wine stock pots are perfect for low-calorie flavouring so there's no need to waste half your day's calorie allowance on wine. This amazing, glossy coq au vin can be served with our French Peas for a total of 390 calories. Mind-blowing!

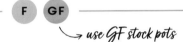

→ *use GF stock pots*

PER SERVING:
282 KCAL
13G CARBS

low-calorie cooking spray
8 small chicken thigh fillets, about 70g each (skin and visible fat removed)
4 bacon medallions, thinly sliced
200g button mushrooms
1 red onion, peeled and roughly chopped
3 garlic cloves, peeled and crushed
1 beef stock pot
2 red wine stock pots
500ml boiling water
2 tbsp tomato puree
2 tsp dried thyme
1 tsp red wine vinegar

TO ACCOMPANY *(optional)*
French Peas, page 226
(+ 108 kcal per serving)

Preheat the oven to 160°C (fan 140°C/gas mark 3).

Place a large casserole dish suitable for both hob and oven onto a high heat. Spray with low-calorie cooking spray and place the chicken into the pan to brown, turning them after 3–4 minutes. Add the sliced bacon medallions and cook for a further 3 minutes. Add all of the remaining ingredients, stir well and put the lid on.

Place in the oven for 1 hour 20 minutes, until the chicken is tender and the sauce has reduced slightly. If the sauce is too thin, remove the lid and pop the dish back into the oven for 5 minutes to reduce it further.

Serve immediately, with your choice of accompaniment. The stew can also be frozen once cooled – defrost fully then reheat until piping hot.

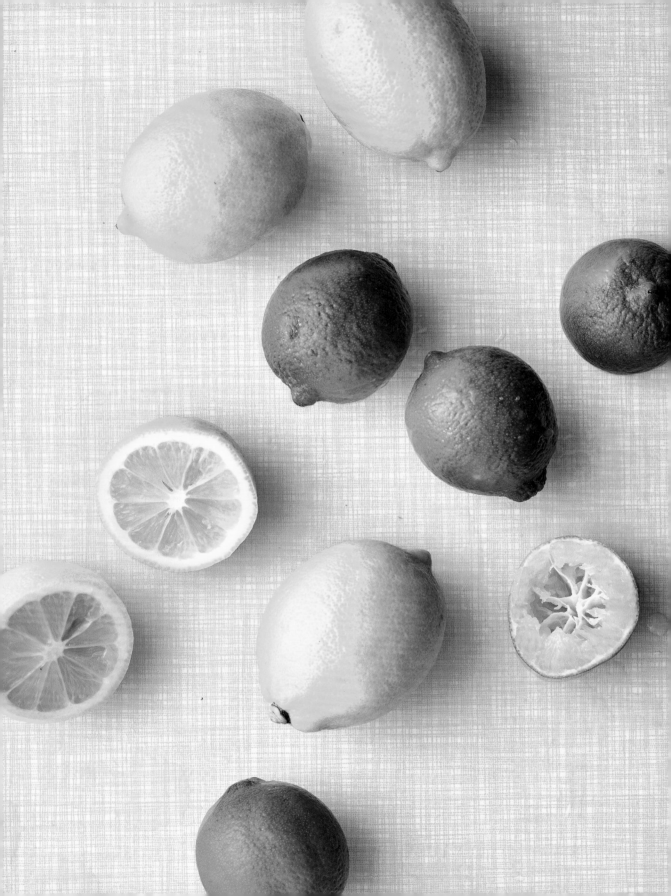

COQ AU VIN

is

ABSOLUTELY

brilliant

JIM

PORK CASSOULET is so *tasty* and really quick to prep. Thanks ladies!

HARRIET

SPRING VEGETABLE SOUP – this is *amazing*!

CAROLINE

SPRING VEGETABLE SOUP

🕐 **15 MINS** | 🍲 **50 MINS** | ✕ **SERVES 4**

This warming soup packs in so many spring veggies, and can be chilled after cooking to use as lunch for the rest of the week. It's so easy to make: just throw everything into the pan and simmer! There's no blending involved in this recipe, keeping the soup chunky and filling.

PER SERVING:
134 KCAL
21G CARBS

low-calorie cooking spray
100g leeks, trimmed, washed
   and thinly sliced
100g carrots, peeled and cut into
   a medium-sized dice
50g celery, cut into a medium-
   sized dice
100g turnip, peeled and cut into
   a medium-sized dice
60g green cabbage, trimmed
   and finely shredded
1.5 litres vegetable stock
   (3 vegetable stock cubes
   dissolved in 1.5 litres
   boiling water)
¼ tsp dried sage
¼ tsp dried thyme
50g barley
100g potatoes, peeled and cut into
   a medium-sized dice
60g frozen peas

Spray a large pan with some low-calorie cooking spray, place over a medium heat, add the leeks, carrots and celery and sauté for 4–5 minutes, until they start to soften. Add the turnip, cabbage, stock, herbs and barley, then bring to the boil. Turn down the heat and simmer for 25 minutes, then add the potato.

Cook for another 20 minutes. Add the peas, then cook for another minute or two. Check the seasoning and serve. The soup can also be frozen once cooled – defrost fully then reheat until piping hot.

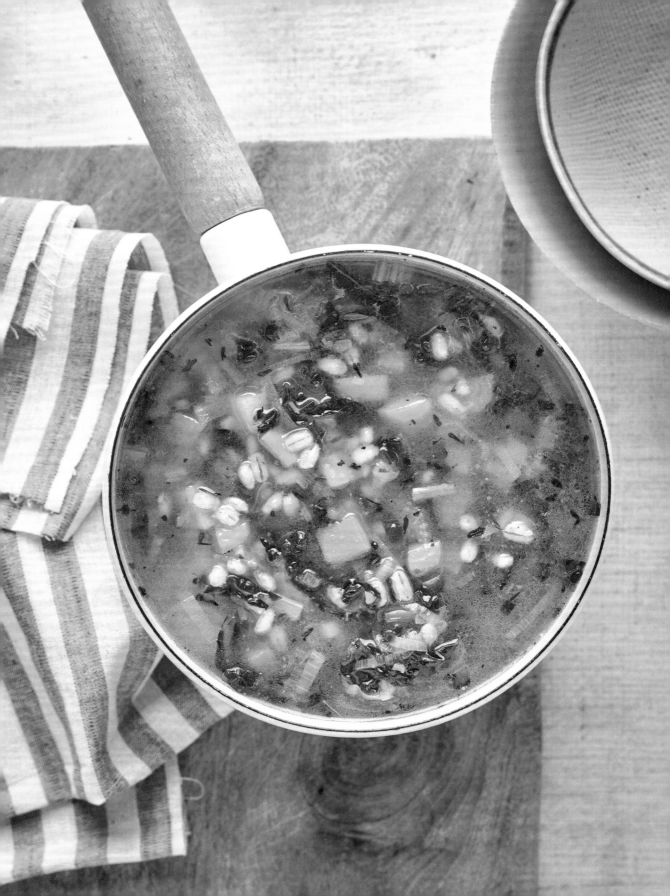

GARLIC, CHICKEN
and RICE SOUP

🕐 **5 MINS** | 🍲 **60 MINS** | ✕ **SERVES 4**

This thick and comforting soup is an absolute winner for when you need a big bowl of something warm and soothing. If you're feeling under the weather, this will sort you right out! If you want to lighten this recipe even more, you can leave out the rice and halve the calories.

PER SERVING:
210 KCAL
32G CARBS

low-calorie cooking spray
2 white onions, peeled and
   roughly chopped
3 garlic cloves, peeled and
   chopped
1 celery stalk, roughly chopped
½ tsp dried tarragon
½ tsp dried thyme
sea salt and freshly ground
   black pepper
1 litre chicken stock (1 chicken
   stock cube dissolved in
   1 litre boiling water)
1 chicken breast, about 165g
   (skin and visible fat removed)
1 head of cauliflower (about
   300g), broken into florets
100g risotto rice or other
   white rice
rosemary sprigs, to garnish
   (optional)

Spray a large saucepan with low-calorie cooking spray and place over a medium heat. Add the onions, garlic and celery and sauté for 5 minutes, until the onions have softened. Add the tarragon, thyme and season with salt and pepper. Stir the mix then pour the stock into the saucepan and add the chicken and cauliflower.

Put the lid on the pan and leave to simmer over a medium–low heat for 40 minutes.

Remove the pan from the heat and take out the chicken breast. Place in a separate bowl and set aside.

Add 250ml of water to the pot and blitz with a stick blender until the soup is smooth. Stir in the rice, replace the lid and put back on a low heat for 15 minutes.

While the rice is cooking, shred the chicken with two forks. When the rice is cooked, stir through the shredded chicken, season with salt and pepper and serve. The soup can also be frozen once cooled – defrost fully then reheat until piping hot.

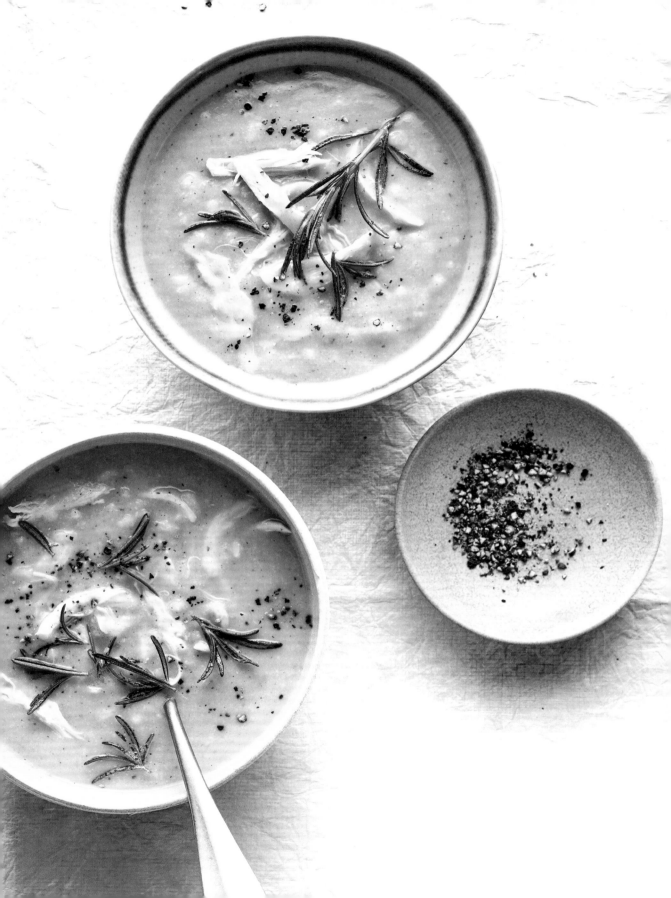

RAMEN BOWLS

🕐 **20 MINS** | 🍲 **30–35 MINS** | ✕ **SERVES 4**

There are many different ways to make Ramen Bowls, but we think our shoyu (soy sauce) version is pretty great! Each portion is full of goodness, packing in six different types of veg. The ginger and chilli give these bowls a kick of flavour, while the chicken and noodles make this meal a filling main.

PER SERVING:
372 KCAL
34G CARBS

200g Tenderstem broccoli
low-calorie cooking spray
1 medium onion, peeled and sliced
2 garlic cloves, peeled and
    finely grated
2.5cm (1in) piece of root ginger,
    peeled and grated
½ fresh chilli, finely chopped (or
    a pinch of dried chilli flakes)
1.2 litres chicken stock (2 chicken
    stock cubes dissoved in
    1.2 litres water)
2 tbsp oyster sauce
3 tbsp rice vinegar
1 tbsp fish sauce
9 tbsp soy sauce
300g chicken breast (skin
    and visible fat removed)
100g spring green cabbage,
    trimmed and shredded
2 nests dry egg noodles

FOR THE TOPPINGS
4 eggs
2 carrots, peeled and cut into thin
    strips (julienne)
1 red pepper, deseeded, thinly sliced
bunch of spring onions, trimmed
    and thinly sliced
lime wedges, to serve (optional)

Trim the florets off the broccoli, place to one side, and thinly slice the remaining stems. Spray a wok with low-calorie cooking spray. Add the onion and broccoli stems and stir-fry for 1 minute.

Add half of the garlic, three-quarters of the ginger, and the chilli, and continue cooking for another minute. Add the stock, oyster sauce, rice vinegar, fish sauce and 8 tablespoons of the soy sauce to the wok and bring to a boil. Add the chicken and reduce the heat to a simmer. Poach the chicken for 15–20 minutes, until it is cooked and there is no pink inside.

Meanwhile, boil the eggs for 7 minutes. While the eggs are boiling, prepare a dish of cold or iced water. When the timer is up, plunge the eggs into the bowl of water. Carefully removed the shells and cut in half.

When the chicken is cooked, remove from the broth and shred. Keep to one side. Add the shredded cabbage to the pan,and cook for 2–3 minutes. Stir-fry the broccoli florets in a separate frying pan or wok with the remaining garlic, and the ginger and soy sauce.

Cook the noodles in a pan of boiling salted water for 4 minutes, then drain.

Assemble the ramen bowls. Evenly distribute the noodles between four bowls. Spoon over the cabbage and broth. Arrange the carrots, pepper, spring onions, shredded chicken and stir-fried broccoli on top. Top each bowl with two egg halves and serve, with lime cheeks for squeezing over (if desired).

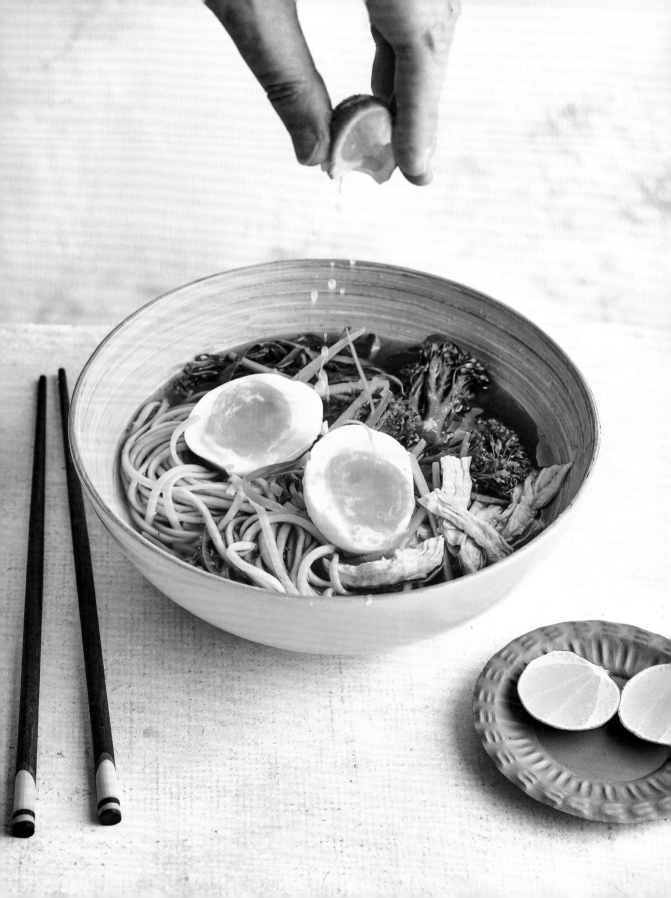

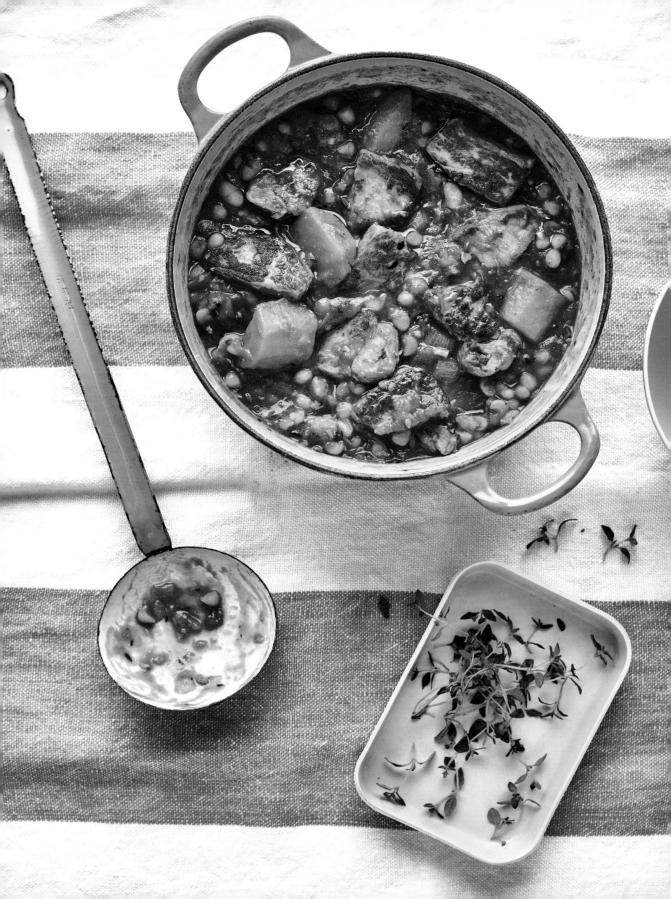

PORK CASSOULET

🕐 **5 MINS** | 🍲 **1 HR 20 MINS** | ✕ **SERVES 6**

Cassoulet is an old dish from the South of France. Made with pork and beans in a hearty sauce, it was a thrifty dish, designed to make meat go further, while still being filling. We've kept all the traditional flavours and ingredients, but cut out all the fat and calories to make this beautifully rich cassoulet.

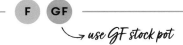

→ *use GF stock pot*

PER SERVING:
222 KCAL
17G CARBS

low-calorie cooking spray
500g lean diced pork
1 large onion, peeled and
    roughly diced
5 garlic cloves, peeled
    and crushed
1 large carrot, peeled and
    thickly sliced
2 tbsp tomato puree
2 tsp fresh or dried thyme
1 tsp fennel seeds
1 x 410g tin haricot beans, drained
350ml vegetable stock
    (1 vegetable stock pot dissolved
    in 350ml boiling water)
1 x 400g tin chopped tomatoes
1 red wine stock pot
fresh thyme (optional)
sea salt and freshly ground
    black pepper

TO ACCOMPANY *(optional)*
Colcannon, page 219 (+ 84 kcal
    per serving)

Preheat the oven to 160°C (fan 140°C/gas mark 3). Place a large, ovenproof, hob-suitable casserole dish onto the hob (the pan should ideally have a lid, but you could cover it with foil), spray with low-calorie cooking spray and brown the pork over a medium heat for 5 minutes.

Add the onion, garlic and carrot to the pan and cook for 3 minutes to soften the veg a little. Add the tomato puree, thyme (if using fresh, just use the leaves, not the stalks) and fennel seeds. Stir well to combine and cook for 2 minutes. Add the remaining ingredients to the pan, season with salt and pepper, and mix. Pop the lid on (or cover the pan with foil) and place in the oven for 35 minutes.

After this, remove the lid, stir and place back in the oven for a further 35 minutes. Serve immediately, with a garnish of fresh thyme if desired. The cassoulet can also be frozen once cooled – defrost fully then reheat until piping hot.

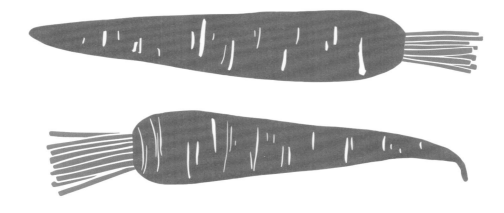

BAKES & ROASTS

RATATOUILLE CHICKEN

🕐 **15–20 MINS** | 🍲 **25 MINS** | ✕ **SERVES 4**

A French dish comprising of vegetables in a rich tomato sauce, this ratatouille is cooked with chicken to give you a very simple, complete meal. Serve with Garlic Scalloped Potatoes for a filling, tasty dinner – just 400 calories for the lot!

F GF

PER SERVING:
224 KCAL
11G CARBS

½ tsp dried basil
1 tsp garlic granules
1 aubergine, trimmed
2 red onions, peeled
2 small courgettes
2 red peppers, deseeded
150g cherry tomatoes
low-calorie cooking spray
4 chicken breasts, about
    150g each (skin and visible
    fat removed)
sea salt and freshly ground
    black pepper
1 tbsp balsamic vinegar
fresh basil leaves, to serve

TO ACCOMPANY (optional)
Garlic Scalloped Potatoes,
    page 234 (+ 176 kcal per serving)

Preheat the oven to 220°C (fan 200°C/gas mark 7).

Mix together the basil and garlic granules and set aside. Cut the vegetables into 1cm (½in)-thick slices and cut the tomatoes in half.

Spray a large casserole dish or oven tray with some low-calorie cooking spray and arrange the sliced vegetables all around the edge of the pan, alternating a slice of aubergine, onion, courgette and pepper.

Place the chicken breasts in the gap in the middle of the veg. Sprinkle the basil and garlic mix over the chicken and veg, season with salt and pepper and spray with some more low-calorie cooking spray.

Place in the oven and cook for 10 minutes. While it is cooking, mix the tomatoes with the balsamic vinegar and season with salt and pepper.

Scatter the tomato mix over the chicken, return to the oven and cook for another 15 minutes, or until the chicken is cooked through. There will be quite a bit of water in the casserole dish after cooking due to the liquid from the veg. Serve scattered with fresh basil. The recipe can also be frozen once cooled – defrost fully then reheat until piping hot.

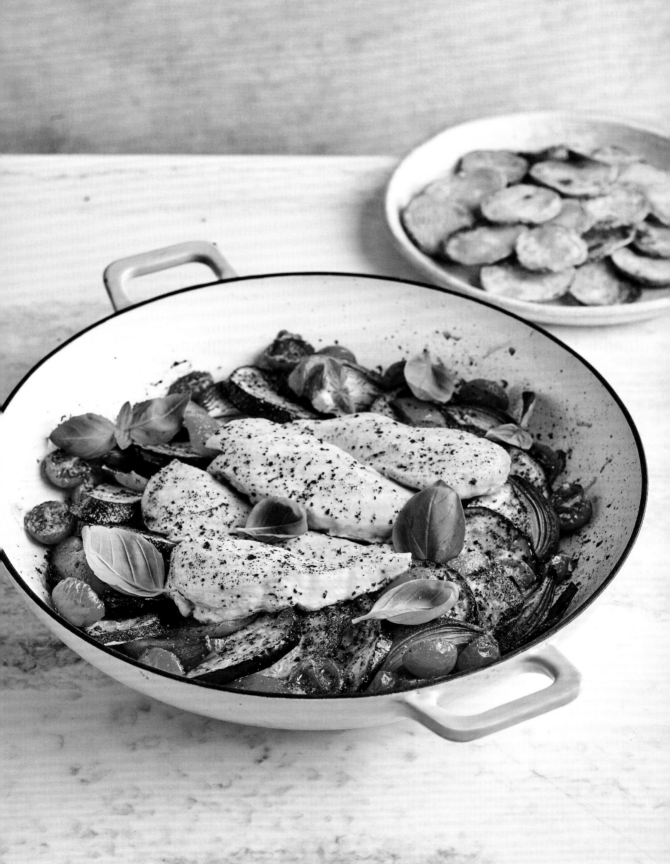

HERB-CRUSTED LAMB

⏱ **5 MINS** | 🍲 **25 MINS** | ✗ **SERVES 4**

Lean lamb can be a little flavourless and dry if you don't pack it full of herbs and spices to enhance the taste. This herby crumb is a great way of adding fresh flavours to the meat and texture along with the breadcrumbs. Garlic, rosemary and lamb are a match made in foodie heaven. This would be a perfect alternative to a roasting joint and would work well with the usual roast-dinner accompaniments, or even rice and vegetables.

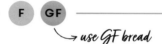
→ use GF bread

PER SERVING:
235 KCAL
6.2G CARBS

4 medium lamb leg steaks
   (about 500g total)
60g wholemeal bread
1 garlic clove, peeled
2 tbsp fresh rosemary leaves
2 tbsp fresh parsley leaves
sea salt and freshly ground
   black pepper
low-calorie cooking spray

TO ACCOMPANY (optional)
Roasted Root Vegetables with
   Garlic and Rosemary, page 247
   (+ 140 kcal per serving)

Preheat the oven to 170°C (fan 150°C/gas mark 3).

Line a baking tray with greaseproof paper. Place the lamb steaks on the baking tray.

Put all of the remaining ingredients (except the salt and pepper and low-calorie cooking spray) into a mini electric chopper or food processor. Blitz into fine breadcrumbs and season with salt and pepper.

Carefully spoon the herby breadcrumbs over the lamb and gently pat down. Spray with low-calorie cooking spray and cook in the oven for 25 minutes until the lamb is cooked and the topping is golden.

Serve with your choice of accompaniment. The lamb can also be frozen once cooled – defrost fully then reheat until piping hot.

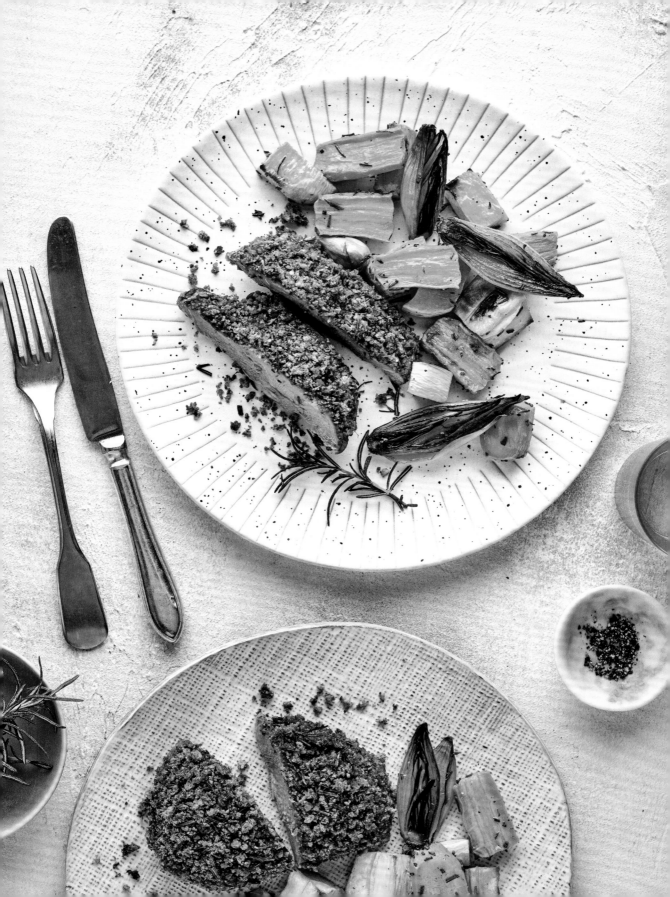

IMAM BAYILDI

🕐 **5 MINS** | 🍲 **40 MINS** | ✗ **SERVES 4**

This Turkish stuffed aubergine dish is traditionally doused in olive oil, and is considered so delicious its name translates as 'The Imam Fainted'. We've reduced the fat and kept things simple, resulting in a dish that can be enjoyed by vegetarians and meat eaters alike, thanks to lemon-flavoured sumac and the other spices. You'll be fainting with shock at it being only 116 calories a portion!

PER SERVING:
116 KCAL
16G CARBS

2 aubergines, sliced lengthways in half
low-calorie cooking spray
sea salt and freshly ground black pepper
2 red onions, peeled and finely chopped
1 red pepper, deseeded and diced
4 garlic cloves, peeled and minced
1 x 400g tin chopped tomatoes
½ tsp sweet paprika
½ tsp sumac (or subsitute 1 tsp lemon juice)
½ tsp ground cinnamon
½ tsp dried oregano
½ tsp granulated sweetener
1 tbsp balsamic vinegar
fresh basil leaves, to serve (optional)

TO ACCOMPANY *(optional)*
50g uncooked rice per portion, cooked according to packet instructions (+ 173 kcal per 125g cooked serving)

Preheat the oven to 220°C (fan 200°C/gas mark 7).

Score the white flesh of the aubergine halves in a criss-cross pattern, without cutting through the skin at the bottom. Spray the halves all over with low-calorie cooking spray and lay on a foil-lined baking tray, cut side up. Season with salt and pepper. Place the tray of aubergine into the middle of the hot oven for 30 minutes.

While the aubergine is cooking, spray a frying pan with low-calorie cooking spray and place over a medium heat. Add the onions, pepper and garlic and sauté for 5 minutes until the onion has softened. Add the tomatoes, paprika, sumac, cinnamon, oregano, sweetener and balsamic vinegar. Season with salt and pepper and simmer for 5 minutes. The mixture will thicken and deepen in colour.

Remove the aubergine halves from the oven. Carefully press down the edges of each aubergine so that the criss-cross sections open up more, creating channels for the sauce to seep into. Spoon the tomato mix on top and place the aubergines back in the oven for 10 minutes.

Remove from the oven and serve. The recipe can also be frozen once cooled. Make sure you defrost thoroughly before reheating in the oven.

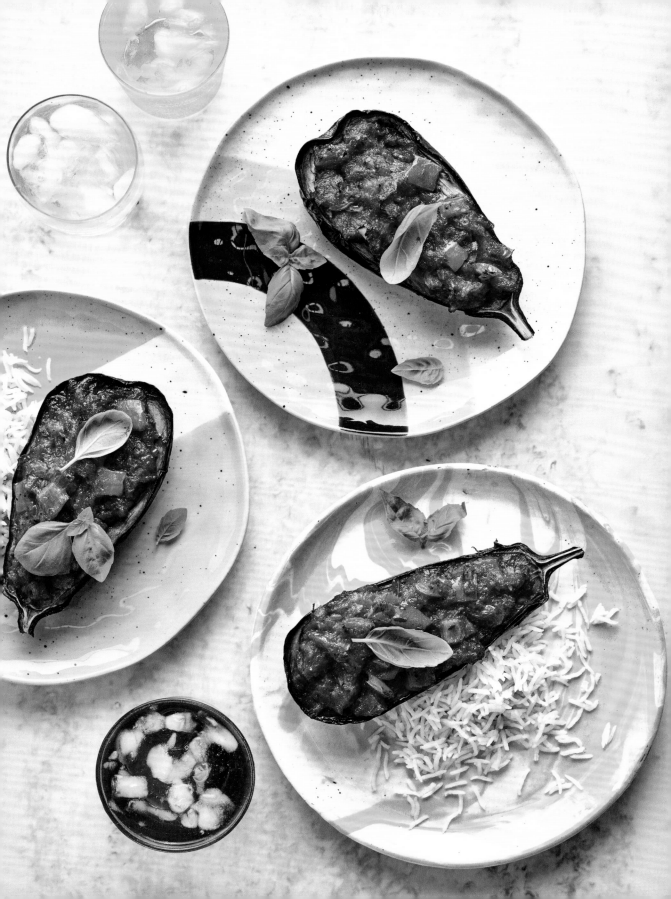

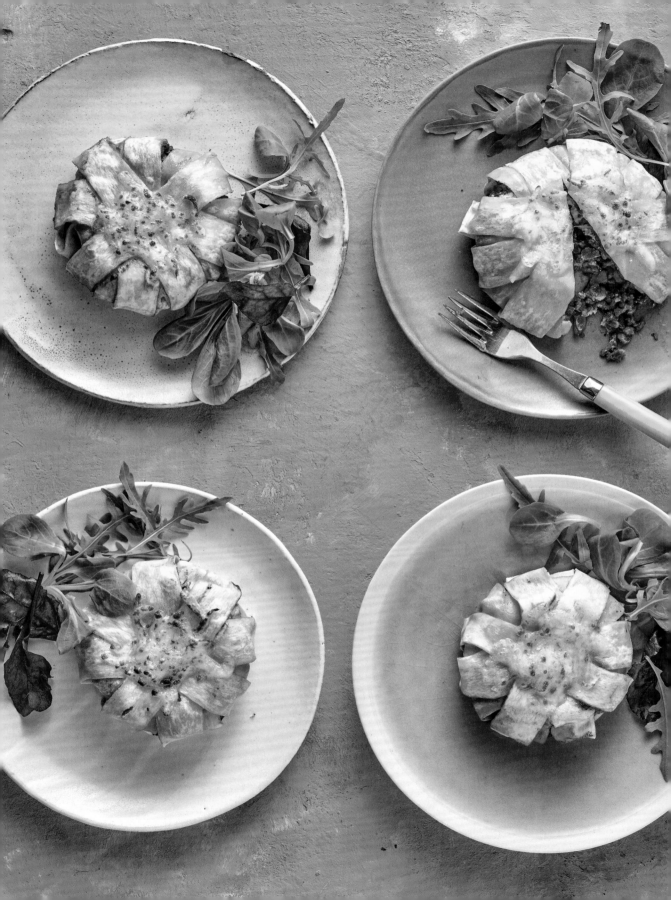

LASAGNE BOWLS

🕐 **10 MINS** | 🍲 **50 MINS** | ✕ **SERVES 4**

This recipe is a great way of serving individual portions of lasagne, but with a twist. There's pasta on the outside, ragu mince in the middle, and an oozy, cheesy centre; lasagne bowls are actually easier to make than a standard lasagne as there's no need to make a cheese sauce: you just need individual (250ml) pudding basins. Serve with a side salad to complete the meal.

F

PER SERVING:
323 KCAL
29G CARBS

low-calorie cooking spray
250g 5%-fat minced beef
1 tomato, very finely diced
4 mushrooms, very finely
  chopped
4 tbsp tomato puree
3 garlic cloves, peeled
  and crushed
2 tsp onion granules
1 tsp dried oregano
1 tsp dried basil
1 beef stock cube
8 dried lasagne sheets (20g each)
40g grated mozzarella
55g light spreadable or
  squeezy cheese

TO ACCOMPANY *(optional)*
75g mixed side salad
  (+ 15 kcal per serving)

MAKE *it* VEGGIE

You could use the Veggie Spaghetti Bolognese recipe on page 144 for an alternative filling.

Spray a large saucepan with low-calorie cooking spray, place over a medium heat, add the minced beef and brown for 5 minutes. Add the fresh tomato, mushrooms, tomato puree, garlic, onion granules, oregano and basil and stir well. Crumble in the stock cube and simmer gently for 25 minutes, until any liquid from the mushrooms and tomato has reduced and you are left with a thick meat ragu.

Meanwhile, bring a large saucepan of water to the boil. Add the lasagne sheets and cook for 5 minutes, gently moving them around the pan to stop them sticking together. Drain, then cut each sheet into four strips, lengthways (each strip will be around 1.5cm (½in wide). Take a 250ml pudding basin and line with the lasagne strips, leaving the excess to overhang the top. The strips should overlap slightly. Repeat with three more pudding basins. Distribute half of the grated mozzarella between the lined pudding basins, setting the other half aside.

Once the meat has finished cooking, add two dessertspoonfuls into each pudding basin. Add a quarter of the spreadable cheese on top, then a further two spoonfuls of meat. Fold over the overhanging pasta to form a lid and place in the oven for 20 minutes until the pasta has cooked through.

Turn out each lasagne bowl onto a baking tray – they may need a little encouragement to come out. Top with the remaining mozzarella and pop under a hot grill for 3–4 minutes or until the cheese is bubbling and turning golden, then serve. The lasagne bowls can also be frozen once cooled – defrost fully then reheat until piping hot.

KEEMA PIE

🕐 **20 MINS** | 🍲 **60 MINS** | ✕ **SERVES 4**

If you love curries and you love pies, then this is the recipe for you! A weekend wonder, this Keema Pie is infused with Indian spices and uses sweet potatoes as well as regular spuds for a mixed mash topping.

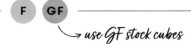

→ use GF stock cubes

PER SERVING:
389 KCAL
52.1G CARBS

FOR THE FILLING
low-calorie cooking spray
400g 5%-fat minced beef
1 onion, peeled and diced
2 bell peppers, deseeded and diced
2 carrots, peeled and diced
1cm (½in) piece of root ginger, peeled and grated
2 tsp garlic granules
2 tbsp curry powder
3 tbsp tomato puree
450ml beef stock (2 beef stock cubes dissolved in 450ml boiling water)
juice of ½ lemon
sea salt and freshly ground black pepper
150g frozen peas

FOR THE TOPPING
500g potatoes (Maris Pipers are ideal)
250g sweet potato
¼ tsp ground turmeric
½ tsp black onion seeds (optional)

Preheat the oven to 200°C (fan 180°C/gas mark 6).

Peel the potatoes and sweet potatoes and cut them into even-sized chunks. Place them in a saucepan, cover with cold salted water and bring to the boil over a high heat. Turn the heat down and allow to simmer for around 20 minutes, or until a knife slides easily into the potatoes.

Meanwhile, cook the mince. Spray a large pan or wok with low-calorie cooking spray, place over a medium–high heat, add the mince and brown for 4–5 minutes. Add the onion, peppers and carrots and continue cooking for another 3–4 minutes. Add the ginger, garlic granules and curry powder. Stir well, then add the tomato puree. Pour in the beef stock, squeeze in the lemon juice, stir well, and bring to the boil.

Reduce the heat to low and allow to simmer uncovered for 20 minutes. The sauce should reduce and thicken. If you think it is a bit runny, cook it for a little longer.

When the potatoes are cooked, drain, return to the pan and mash well. Add the turmeric and onion seeds if using, and mix in. Taste and add salt and pepper as necessary.

When the mince is cooked, stir through the frozen peas, then place the mix into a deep ovenproof dish. A lasagne dish is perfect. (At this point you could allow it to cool completely and freeze for topping and baking at a later date.)

Once the filling has cooled slightly, spread the mashed potatoes on top of the meat and fluff up with a fork. Place in the preheated oven for 30 minutes, or until the topping is golden.

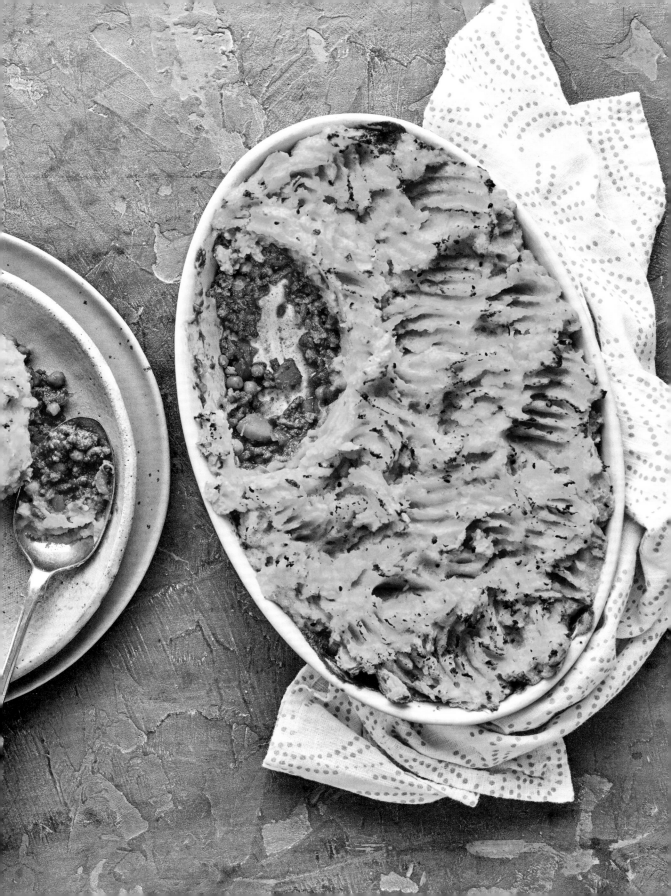

ZA'ATAR CHICKEN

🕐 **15 MINS** (PLUS MARINATING TIME) | 🍲 **35 MINS** | ✕ **SERVES 4**

Za'atar is a fragrant spice mix originating from the Middle East and it tastes amazing when used to flavour chicken. This recipe is a great one to serve when having dinner with friends, as it's so quick and easy to make. You can guarantee that your guests will be going back for seconds!

PER SERVING:
371 KCAL
34G CARBS

4 medium chicken breasts, about 165g each (skin and visible fat removed)
500g new potatoes, washed and halved
1 red pepper, deseeded and cut into large dice
1 red onion, peeled and cut into large chunks
juice of ½ lemon
1 tsp sesame seeds
sea salt and freshly ground black pepper

FOR THE SPICE MARINADE
2 tsp sumac
½ tsp dried thyme
½ tsp dried oregano
½ tsp garlic granules
3 tbsp fat-free natural yoghurt

FOR THE YOGHURT AND MINT DRESSING
8 tbsp fat-free natural yoghurt
1 tsp mint sauce

Preheat the oven to 200°C (fan 180°C/gas mark 6).

Mix the marinade ingredients together in a bowl, then coat the chicken breasts. Cover and marinate for 30 minutes.

Bring a pan of salted water to the boil and add the new potatoes. Simmer for 10 minutes, then drain well.

Spray a baking sheet with low-calorie cooking spray, mix the potatoes with the pepper and onion and spread out evenly on the tray. Place the chicken breasts on top. Pour over the lemon juice, sprinkle over the sesame seeds, season with salt and pepper and bake in the oven for 25 minutes until the chicken is cooked and there is no pink left in the middle.

Mix the remaining yoghurt with the teaspoon of mint sauce in a bowl.

Divide the chicken and vegetables between four plates, drizzle with the yoghurt dressing and serve.

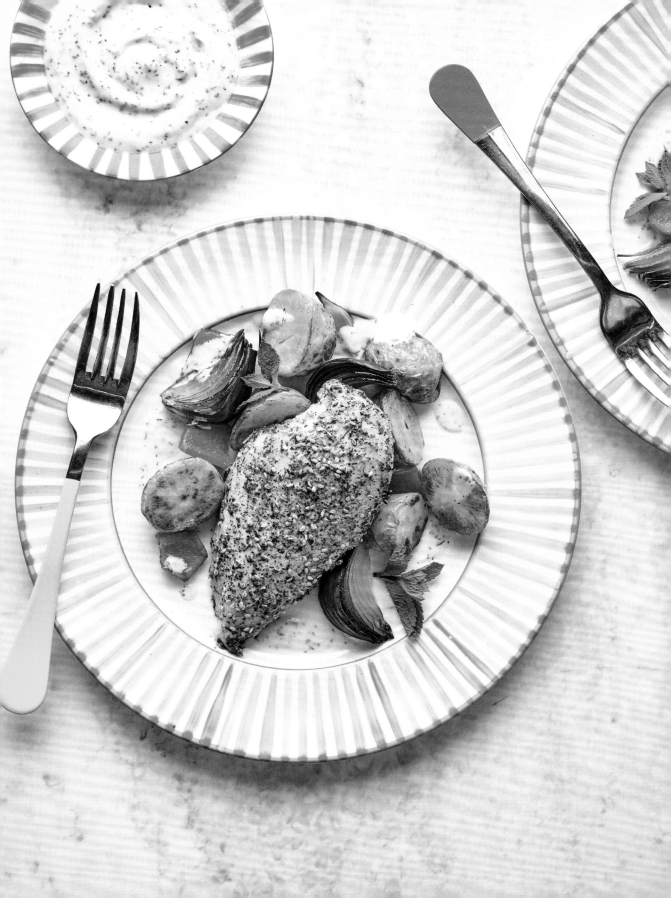

CREAMY VEGETABLE BAKE

🕐 **5 MINS** | 🍲 **45 MINS** | ✗ **SERVES 4**

This recipe is a great way of using up any small amounts of vegetables and brings them all together in a creamy, cheesy sauce. You can use whatever veg you have – root vegetables work particularly well. The breadcrumbs on top add some crunch to the texture. Serve on its own or as a side dish.

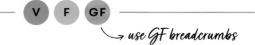

V **F** **GF**

↳ use GF breadcrumbs

PER SERVING:
340 KCAL
30G CARBS

low-calorie cooking spray
1 small sweet potato, scrubbed
   and cut into roughly 2cm
   (¾ in) chunks (about 130g)
2 small leeks, trimmed,
   washed and cut into roughly
   2cm (¾ in) chunks
1 small carrots, peeled and cut into
   roughly 2cm (¾ in) chunks
2 small parsnips, peeled and cut
   into roughly 2cm (¾ in) chunks
200g cauliflower, trimmed and
   broken into florets
360g ricotta
220g light spreadable or
   squeezy cheese
2 tsp mustard powder
sea salt and freshly ground
   black pepper
60g wholemeal bread

TO ACCOMPANY *(optional)*
75g mixed side salad
   (+ 15 kcal per serving)

Preheat the oven to 160°C (fan 140°C/gas mark 3).

Spray the base of a large ovenproof baking dish with low-calorie cooking spray and add the vegetables.

In a jug, combine the ricotta, spreadable cheese, mustard powder, 200ml water, and a pinch each of salt and pepper. Mix well. Pour over the vegetables and stir to ensure a good coating.

Place the bread in a mini electric chopper or food processor and blitz into fine crumbs. Spread the breadcrumbs over the vegetables to form an even coating. Pop in the oven and cook until the top is golden and the veg are just tender – this will take between 35–45 minutes. Take out and serve while hot. The bake can also be frozen once cooled – defrost fully then reheat until piping hot.

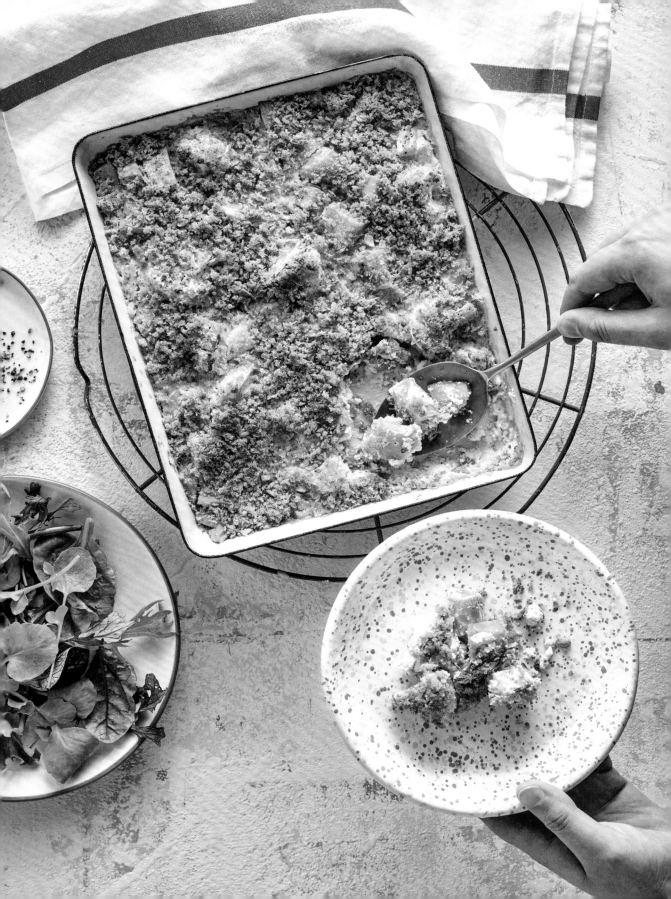

LEEK *and* BACON TARTIFLETTE

🕐 **10 MINS** | 🍲 **50 MINS** | 🍴 **SERVES 4**

Tartiflette is a dish from the Alps, usually containing potatoes, cheese, bacon and onions. We've added a leeky twist to this recipe and used reduced-fat Cheddar and quark to keep it slimming-friendly without compromising on the traditional flavours. This is such a comforting dinner to come home to and is guaranteed to warm the cockles!

F **GF**

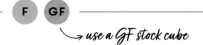 *→ use a GF stock cube*

PER SERVING:
349 KCAL
38G CARBS

650g potatoes, washed and diced, (no need to peel)
low-calorie cooking spray
1 small red onion, peeled and diced
350g leeks, trimmed, washed and thinly sliced
350g bacon medallions, diced
2 tsp garlic granules
1 tsp mustard powder
60g spinach
200ml chicken stock (1 chicken stock cube dissolved in 200ml boiling water)
110g light spreadable or squeezy cheese
100g quark
80g reduced-fat Cheddar, grated
sea salt and freshly ground black pepper

MAKE *it* VEGGIE

Omit the bacon or replace it with quorn bacon-style rashers or slices

Preheat the oven to 220°C (fan 200°C/gas mark 7).

Put the diced potatoes into a pan of water and bring to the boil on the hob. Turn the heat down and simmer until they are cooked through, but be careful not to overcook them; they still need to hold their shape well. This should take about 15 minutes. When they are cooked, remove them from the heat and drain.

Spray a frying pan with low-calorie cooking spray, then add the onion and leeks and sauté over a medium heat for 3–4 minutes, until they start to soften. Add the bacon, 1 teaspoon of the garlic granules and the mustard powder. Continue to cook for around 10 minutes. Add the spinach and cook until it has lightly wilted.

Pour in the stock and cook for 2 minutes. Stir in the spreadable cheese, then remove the pan from the heat. Make a well in the centre of the mixture and add the quark. To prevent the quark from splitting, work from the centre out until fully combined. Season with salt and pepper to taste.

If your frying pan isn't suitable for the oven, transfer the mixture to an ovenproof dish. Sprinkle half the cheese over the top evenly, then cover with the cooked potato. Sprinkle the remaining garlic granules over the top, season then cook in the oven for 15 minutes.

Sprinkle the remaining cheese over the top and return to the oven for another 15 minutes until the cheese has melted and started to colour. Remove from the oven and serve. The recipe can also be frozen once cooled.

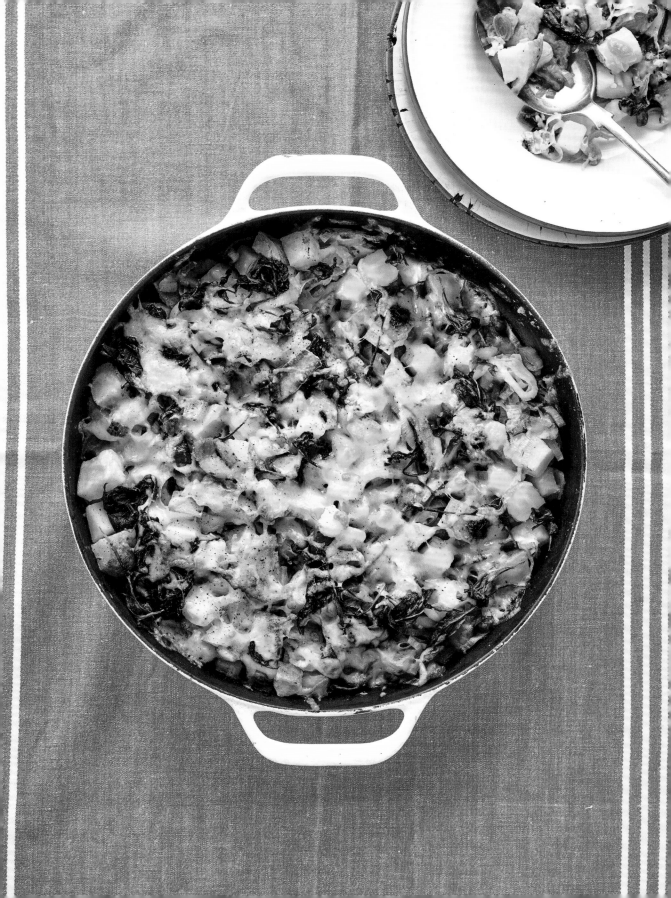

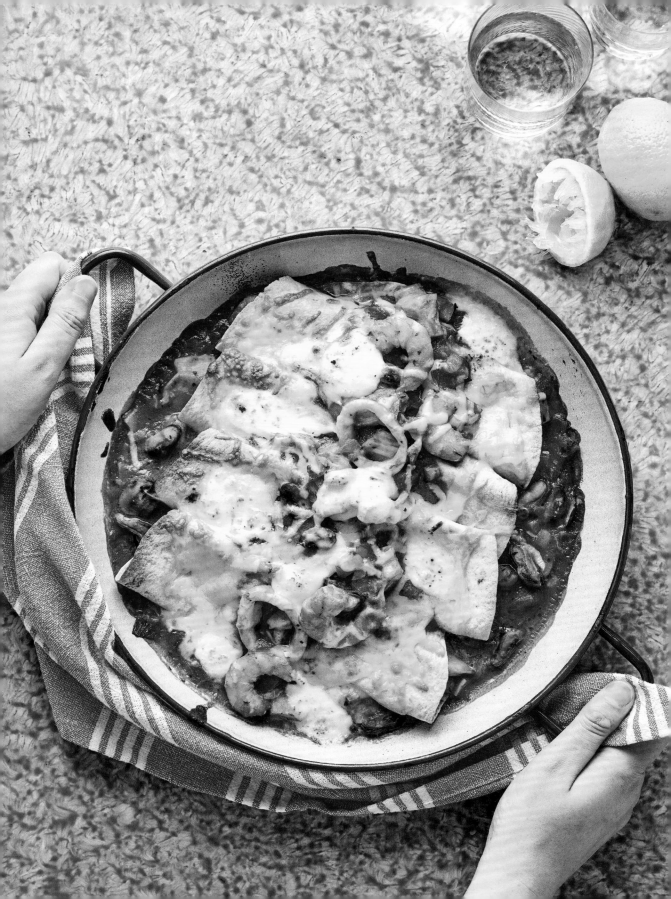

SEAFOOD CRESPELLA

⏱ **15 MINS** | 🍲 **50 MINS** | ✗ **SERVES 4**

A Seafood Crespella is ordinarily a dish made with crepes, packed with seafood and rolled up like enchiladas with a cheesy, cream-filled sauce on top. Of course, we put the Pinch of Nom twist on this and switched the crepes for low-calorie tortillas and brought the calories right down by using clever ingredient swaps and removing the oils and fats of the original. Tasty but healthy – smashed it!

F

→ use raw seafood mix

PER SERVING:
370 KCAL
35G CARBS

low-calorie cooking spray
1 red onion, peeled and diced
1 red or yellow pepper, deseeded
    and diced
2 garlic cloves, peeled and
    crushed
60g mushrooms, sliced
¼ tsp dried Italian herbs
1 tsp balsamic vinegar
1 x 500g carton passata
200g fresh salmon
200g seafood mix (raw or cooked)
1 fish stock pot
sea salt and freshly ground
    black pepper
4 low-fat tortilla wraps
40g reduced-fat Cheddar, grated
70g reduced-fat mozzarella
paprika (optional)

TO ACCOMPANY *(optional)*
75g mixed side salad
    (+ 15 kcal per serving)

Preheat the oven to 160°C (fan 140°C/gas mark 3).

Spray a frying pan with some low-calorie cooking spray, then place over a medium heat, add the onion, pepper and garlic and sauté for 4–5 minutes until soft but not coloured.

Add the mushrooms, herbs and balsamic vinegar and cook for another 2 minutes. Stir in the passata, then turn the heat down and simmer for 10 minutes.

Add the raw salmon, seafood mix (if you're using raw) and the fish stock pot, cook for 5 minutes. If you're using cooked seafood mix add it after the 5 minutes and stir well. Taste and add some salt and pepper if necessary.

Put a couple of spoonfuls of the sauce and seafood mix into the bottom of an ovenproof dish, then fill each wrap with the sauce and seafood mix and roll them loosely. Keep a couple of spoonfuls of the mix aside.

Place the filled wraps in the dish with the join on the bottom. Put the remaining sauce and seafood mix over the top, then sprinkle the grated Cheddar evenly over the top. Tear the mozzarella into pieces and sprinkle evenly over the top. If you want, you can sprinkle over a little paprika to add some extra colour.

Cook in the oven for around 25 minutes, until the cheese is melted and golden. This bake can also be frozen once cooled – defrost fully then reheat until piping hot.

LENTIL *and* ROOT VEGETABLE BAKE

🕐 **15 MINS** | 🍲 **1 HR 5 MINS** | ✕ **SERVES 4**

Lentils are perfect for a meat-free alternative in bakes and pies, as they are high in protein and fibre so help keep you feeling full until your next meal. This recipe uses a splodge of Marmite to add depth to the flavour of the stock. Using cooking spray on the potatoes and swede before they go into the oven is a great way of making sure they crisp up nicely, without the need for lots of oil.

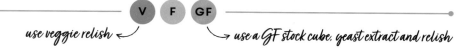

use veggie relish ← **V** **F** **GF** → *use a GF stock cube, yeast extract and relish*

PER SERVING:
305 KCAL
49G CARBS

400g potatoes, peeled and cut
    into large chunks
1 small swede (about 400g),
    peeled
140g green lentils
low-calorie cooking spray
1 onion, peeled and finely chopped
2 garlic cloves, peeled
    and minced
1 tsp dried thyme
1 tbsp tomato puree
1 tsp Marmite or GF yeast extract
100ml vegetable stock
    (1 vegetable stock cube
    dissolved in 100ml boiling water)
1 x 400g tin chopped tomatoes
1 tbsp Henderson's relish
    or Worcestershire sauce
2 carrots, peeled and grated
sea salt and freshly ground
    black pepper

Preheat the oven to 200°C (fan 180°C/gas mark 6).

Place the potatoes and swede in a large pan of salted water, bring to the boil and cook for 5 minutes. Drain and place to one side to cool.

Place the lentils in a sieve or colander and give them a good rinse. Transfer to a saucepan, cover with plenty of water, and bring to a rapid boil. Turn down the heat and simmer gently for 20 minutes.

While the lentils are simmering, spray a saucepan with low-calorie cooking spray, place over a medium heat, add the onion andd sauté for 3–4 minutes, until soft. Add the garlic, thyme and tomato puree and stir well. Dissolve the Marmite in the stock and add this to the pan along with the chopped tomatoes and Henderson's relish. Stir in the grated carrot and bring to a gentle boil. Reduce the heat and simmer for 10 minutes.

Add the cooked lentils, stir well, taste and season with salt and pepper. Pour the lentil mix into an ovenproof dish.

Now, coarsely grate the part-cooked potato and swede into a large bowl, season with salt and pepper and mix well. Scatter the potato and swede mix evenly over the lentils, spray the top with low-calorie cooking spray, and place in the preheated oven. Cook for 25–30 minutes, so that the centre of the rosti topping is soft and the top is golden. This bake can also be frozen once cooled – defrost fully then reheat until piping hot.

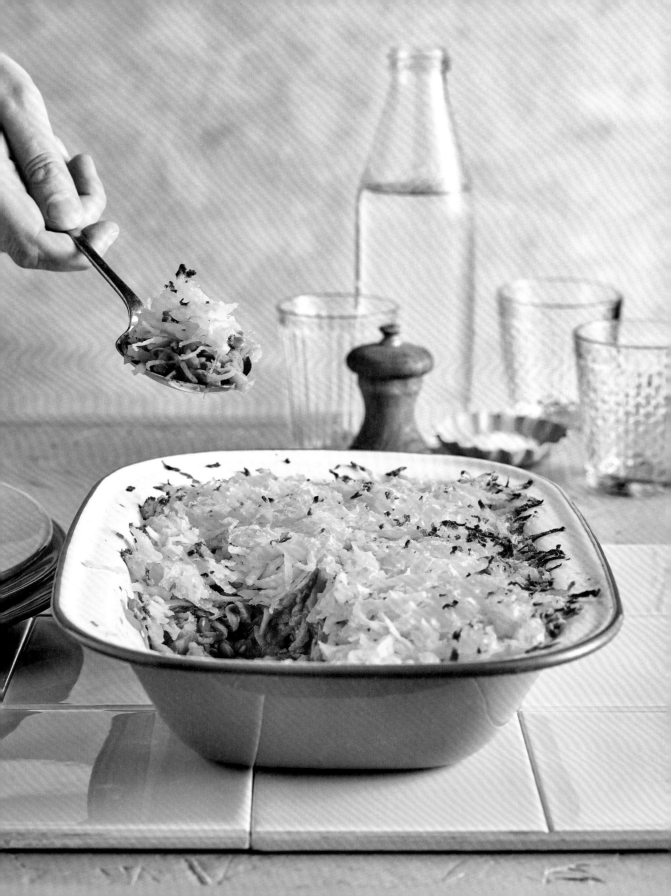

MOUSSAKA CANNELLONI

🕐 **15 MINS** | 🍲 **60 MINS** | ✕ **SERVES 6**

A twist on the classic moussaka, this Greek-inspired dish doesn't actually contain any pasta! The 'cannelloni' are made from aubergines, rolled into tubes stuffed with a meaty filling and topped with our lower-calorie take on a béchamel sauce. Traditional Greek flavours minus the calories will have you thinking you're on holiday in no time! (Pictured overleaf.)

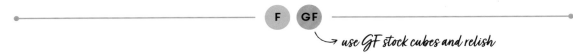

F GF

→ *use GF stock cubes and relish*

PER SERVING:
358 KCAL
29.4G CARBS

FOR THE MEAT SAUCE
low-calorie cooking spray
3 onions, peeled and finely diced
2 carrots, peeled and finely diced
2 celery sticks, finely diced
2 red peppers, deseeded and
　finely diced
2 courgettes, finely diced
1 tsp dried mint
2 tsp dried oregano
2 tsp dried basil
4 garlic cloves, peeled and minced
500g 5%-fat minced beef
sea salt and freshly ground
　black pepper
200ml lamb stock (2 lamb stock
　cubes dissolved in 200ml
　boiling water)
1 red wine stock pot
1 x 400g tin chopped tomatoes
3 large aubergines, cut lengthways
　into 5mm (¼ in)-thick slices
6 tbsp tomato puree
1 tbsp balsamic vinegar
2 tsp Worcestershire sauce
　or Henderson's relish

Preheat the oven to 220°C (fan 200°C/gas mark 7).

Spray a saucepan with low-calorie cooking spray. Add the onions, carrots and celery to the pan and sauté over a medium heat for 10 minutes, until the carrot has softened and the onions start to turn translucent. Add the peppers and courgettes to the pan with the mint, oregano, basil and garlic. Add the mince to the saucepan, season with salt and pepper and stir. Cook for 5 minutes, until the mince has browned.

Add the lamb stock to the pan and stir in the red wine stock pot. Stir in the chopped tomatoes and place a lid on. Leave to simmer for 15 minutes while you are preparing the aubergine.

Place the slices of aubergine on a baking tray. Place at the bottom of the hot oven for 15 minutes. They should dry out and now be easier to roll. This will allow you to shape them later and prevent too much water pooling in the bottom of your dish.

When the meat sauce in the saucepan has finished cooking, stir in the tomato puree, balsamic vinegar and Worcestershire sauce. The sauce should be very thick and rich; if it's still a little runny, reduce for a few minutes with the lid off. Then take off the heat and let it cool for a few minutes more.

FOR THE WHITE SAUCE

300g fat-free Greek yoghurt

1 egg

½ tsp onion granules

½ tsp garlic granules

¼ tsp ground nutmeg

¼ tsp ground cinnamon

120g reduced-fat Cheddar,
   finely grated

TO ACCOMPANY *(optional)*

75g mixed side salad
   (+ 15 kcal per serving)

While the meat sauce is cooling, make the white sauce. Mix the Greek yoghurt, egg, onion granules, garlic granules, nutmeg and cinnamon in a separate bowl until smooth. Season with salt and pepper and set aside.

Now begin assembling the dish. Roll a slice of the aubergine and place in a roasting dish so that you can see down to the bottom of the tray like a tube. Spoon a few tablespoons of the meat sauce in and repeat until the dish is filled with the aubergine and meat tubes (pictured on page 196). Spoon the white sauce onto the top of the tubes and sprinkle over the Cheddar.

Bake in the oven for 25 minutes. The top of the sauce should be set and the cheese will be bubbling. Remove from the oven and serve. The moussaka can also be frozen once cooled – defrost fully then reheat until piping hot.

Tip

If you want to speed this dish up a little, you can layer the aubergine slices as you would with pasta in a lasagne. This will make it more like a traditional moussaka.

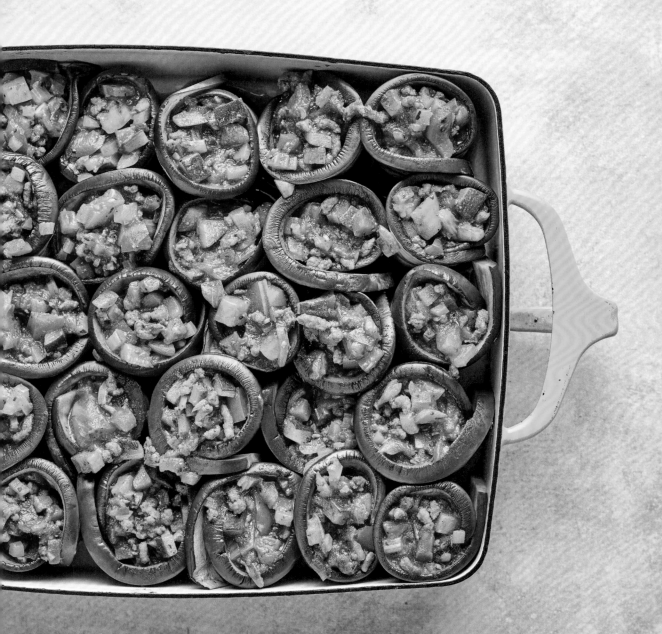

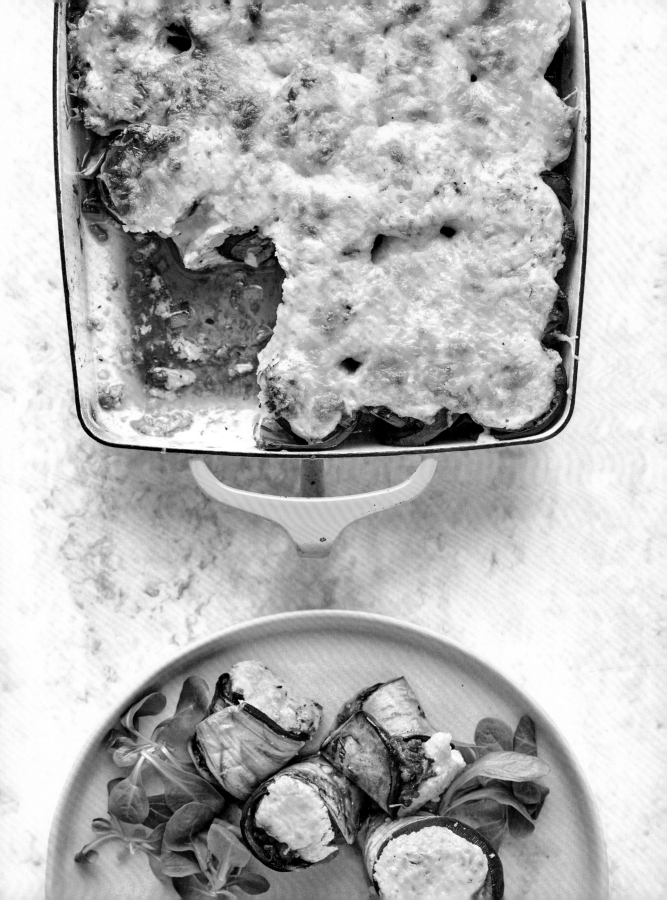

PIRI PIRI
ROAST CHICKEN

🕐 **10 MINS** | 🍲 **ABOUT 1 HR 30 MINS** | ✕ **SERVES 6**

Here's traditional roast chicken with a spicy makeover. It's hard to believe that you can pack so many flavours into one roast chicken, but here we've put our Pinch of Nom spin on things! We recommend removing the skin before eating, but no added oils or fats means you can indulge occasionally. You could also serve with Batatas Picantes (see page 250) for a treat if you don't mind the extra calories.

GF

PER SERVING:
294 KCAL
1G CARBS

1 large chicken
2 limes, halved
2–3 medium-sized red chillies, deseeded
1 tsp hot chilli powder (or medium hot, if you prefer less heat)
3 garlic cloves, peeled
1 tsp onion salt
1 tsp paprika
½ tsp granulated sweetener or sugar
½ tsp dried oregano
½ tsp ground coriander
2 tsp red wine vinegar
small handful of fresh oregano (optional)
50ml water

TO ACCOMPANY *(optional)*
75g mixed side salad
  (+ 15 kcal per serving)

Around 30 minutes before you wish to cook, take the chicken out of the fridge.

Preheat the oven to 190°C (fan 170°C/gas mark 5).

Squeeze the lime juice into a small dish and set the remaining pith and peel aside for later. Place the juice, along with all the remaining ingredients, apart from the chicken, water and the fresh oregano, in a blender and blitz until it forms a paste.

Rub the paste all over the chicken, making sure to rub some between the skin and the breast meat. (To do this, loosen the skin from the breast by sliding your fingers between the meat and the skin from either end of the chicken.)

Cut the remains of one of the limes into four pieces and lay on the bottom of a roasting tin or tray. Stuff the remaining lime pith and peel inside the chicken cavity, along with the fresh oregano, if you're using it. Place the chicken on top of the limes, add the water to the tray and cook according to the packaging instructions. The chicken will be cooked when the juices run clear when you insert a knife into the thickest part of the leg. (This should take roughly 40 minutes per kilo, plus an extra 20 minutes.)

Remove from the oven and leave to rest for 15 minutes before serving.

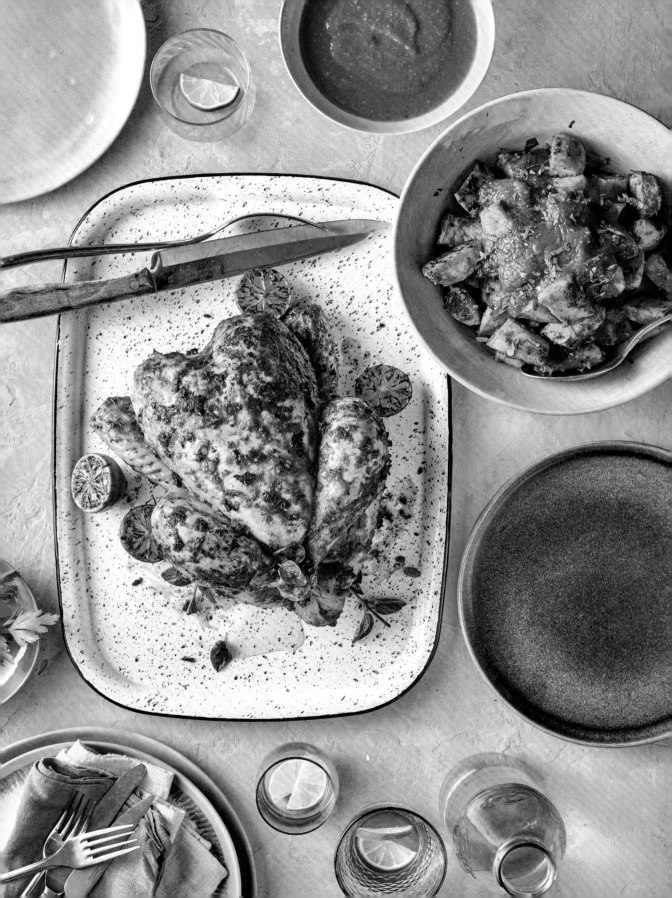

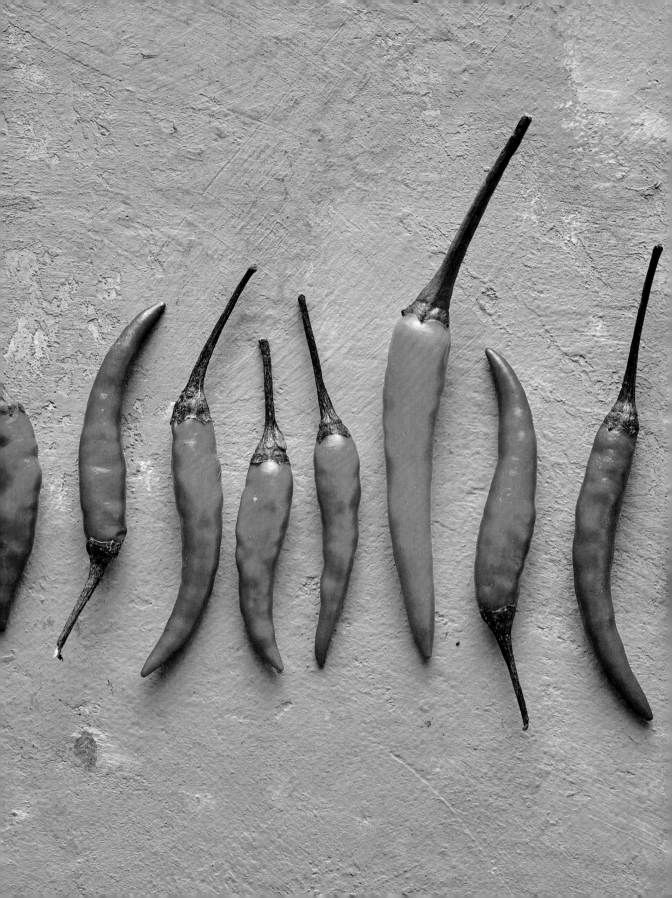

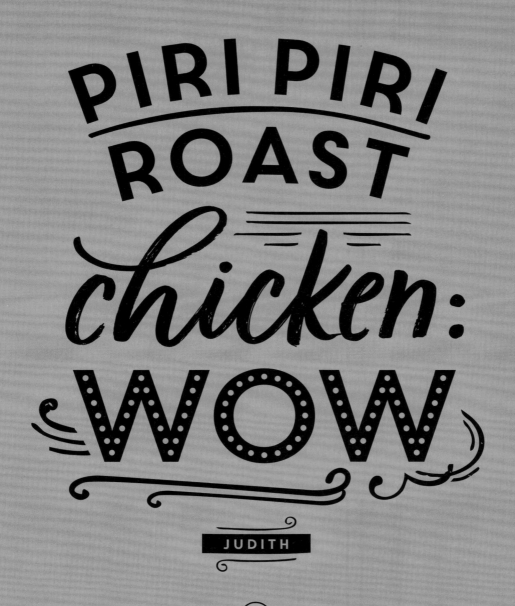

PIRI PIRI ROAST chicken: WOW

JUDITH

> **RATATOUILLE CHICKEN** went down a *treat* and was so easy to make.
>
> CHELSEA

> I could have had the *whole* **LENTIL AND ROOT VEGETABLE BAKE** to myself.
>
> SHIRLEY

SPINACH, FETA *and* POTATO BAKE

🕐 **15 MINS** | 🍲 **1 HR 30 MINS** | ✕ **SERVES 4**

This vegetarian potato bake uses only a few ingredients and is so easy to make, but will taste as if you've been gourmet cooking for an afternoon! Spinach and feta is a simple yet delicious flavour combination and this meal is a real treat to serve without the calories. Serve with a side salad or steamed vegetables.

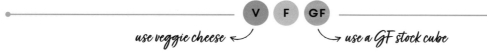

use veggie cheese ↙   ↘ *use a GF stock cube*

PER SERVING:
306 KCAL
47G CARBS

low-calorie cooking spray
½ red onion, peeled and
    finely chopped
1 garlic clove, peeled and chopped
250g spinach
juice of 1 lemon
1kg potatoes, peeled and
    thinly sliced
130g reduced-fat feta or Greek
    salad cheese
200ml vegetable stock
    (1 vegetable stock cube dissolved
    in 200ml boiling water)
sea salt and freshly ground
    black pepper

Preheat the oven to 180°C (fan 160°C/gas mark 4).

Spray a large frying pan with low-calorie cooking spray, place over a medium heat, add the onion and sauté for 2–3 minutes, until soft. Add the garlic and spinach to the pan with half the lemon juice and continue to cook until the spinach wilts.

Spray an ovenproof dish with low-calorie cooking spray. Place one third of the sliced potatoes in the bottom of the dish, top with half the spinach mix, then crumble half of the feta on top. Add another layer of potatoes, spinach and feta, and then top with the remaining potato.

Mix the remaining lemon juice into the stock, pour over the potatoes, and season the top with salt and pepper to taste. Cover with foil and place in the oven for 1 hour.

After an hour, remove the foil and check. Add a little water if it has dried out. Return to the oven, uncovered, for 15–30 minutes. The remaining cooking time will depend on how thick you have sliced the potatoes. They are cooked when golden on top and a knife slides easily into the middle of the potato bake. The bake can also be frozen once cooled – defrost fully then reheat until piping hot.

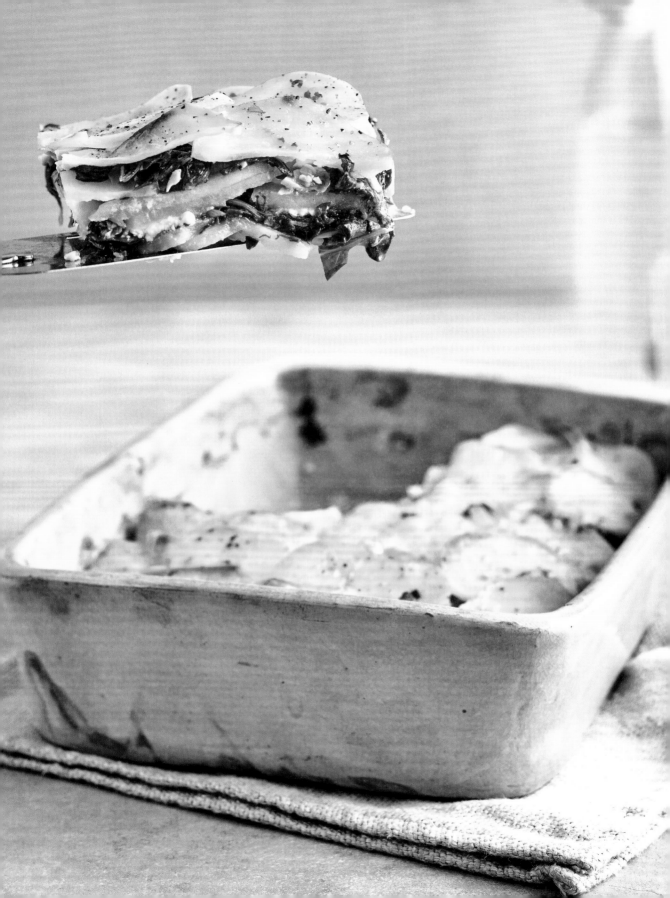

ROOTS ROSTI

⏱ **10 MINS** | 🍲 **40 MINS** | ✕ **SERVES 4**

This recipe uses some favourite root vegetables, plus some simple flavours, all bound together with egg and the magic ingredient that is xanthan gum. This gluten-free powder helps bind things together, and a little goes a long way. You could add any root veg you like!

PER SERVING:
127 KCAL
14G CARBS

1 small swede, peeled
1 small sweet potato, scrubbed
1 small carrot, peeled
1 small parsnip, peeled
low-calorie cooking spray
2 large eggs
1 tsp onion granules
1 tsp garlic granules
1 tsp xanthan gum
sea salt and freshly ground
    black pepper

TO ACCOMPANY *(optional)*
Poached egg and Ketchup
    Tomatoes, page 221
    (+ 92 kcal per serving)

Preheat the oven to 180°C (fan 160°C/gas mark 4) and line a baking tray with greaseproof paper.

Finely grate all of the root vegetables into a large bowl, lined with a clean tea towel. Gather up the corners of the tea towel and, over a sink, squeeze all the liquid out of the grated vegetables. Return the vegetables to a large bowl and mix in all the remaining ingredients, seasoning with salt and pepper.

Place an 8cm (3¼ in) crumpet ring onto the baking tray and add two large dessertspoonfuls of the vegetables into the ring. Press down with the back of the spoon and gently remove the crumpet ring. Each rosti should measure about 1.5cm (½in) in height. Repeat until you have made twelve rostis.

Spray each rosti with low-calorie cooking spray and place in the oven for 40 minutes, flipping carefully when it is firm enough to fip over (roughtly after 20–25 minutes cooking) and spraying again with low-calorie cooking spray. Serve straight from the oven. The rosti can also be frozen once cooled – defrost fully before reheating.

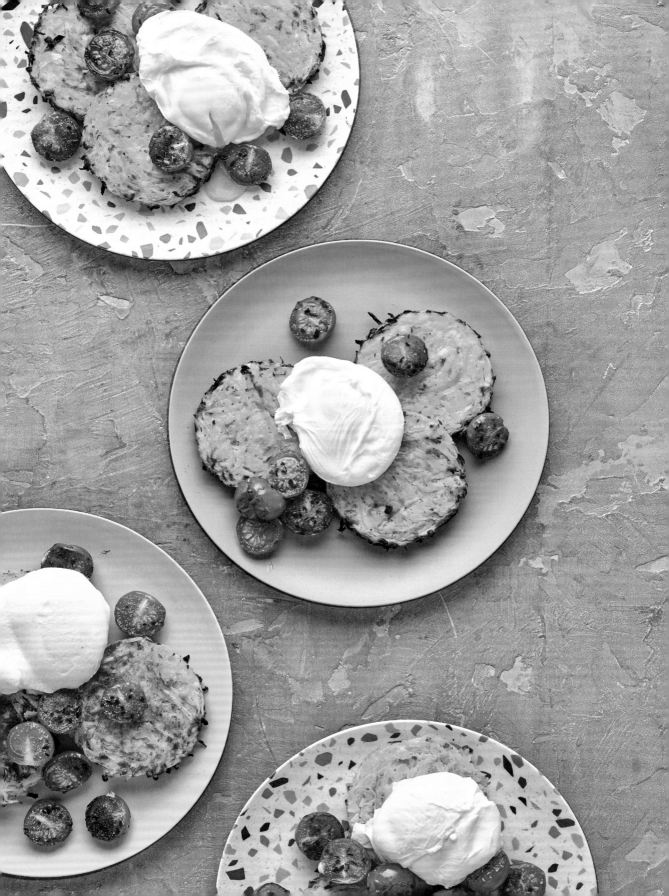

PASTITSIO

⏱ **10 MINS** | 🍲 **55 MINS** | ✕ **SERVES 8**

The traditional version of this Greek dish can be time-consuming to cook, with layers of ground meat and béchamel sauce. Our version is made up of just two layers; meaty sauce and pasta on the bottom, white sauce and pasta on top. This is a lot easier than the traditional method but still retains the delicious, authentic flavours! Serve with mixed salad if you don't mind the extra 15 calories per portion.

F

PER SERVING:
400 KCAL
53G CARBS

1 celery stick
3 carrots, peeled
3 large white onions, peeled
low-calorie cooking spray
6 garlic cloves, peeled and minced
400g 5%-fat minced beef
1 beef stock cube
1 red wine stock pot
200ml boiling water
300g mushrooms (about 15)
1 tsp dried thyme
½ tsp ground cinnamon
1 tbsp balsamic vinegar
1 tbsp Worcestershire sauce
   or Henderson's relish
sea salt and freshly ground
   black pepper
2 x 400g tins chopped tomatoes
375g pasta (we used macaroni)
1 x 500g carton passata
2 tbsp tomato puree

FOR THE WHITE SAUCE
500g fat-free Greek yoghurt
2 eggs
½ tsp ground nutmeg
1 tsp onion granules
1 tsp garlic granules

Preheat the oven to 200°C (fan 180°C/gas mark 6).

Finely chop the celery, carrots and onions and add to a saucepan with the low-calorie cooking spray and the minced garlic. Sauté over a medium heat for about 5 minutes until softened. Add the minced beef and brown for about 5 minutes.

Add the stock cube and wine stock pot to the 200ml boiling water and dissolve. Pour the stock into the saucepan. Finely chop or dice the mushrooms and add them to the pan along with the thyme, cinnamon, balsamic vinegar, Worcestershire sauce. Season with salt and pepper and simmer for about 5 minutes.

Add the chopped tomatoes then put the lid on the pan and leave to simmer over a low heat for about 15 minutes.

Meanwhile, cook the pasta according to the packet instructions. While the pasta is cooking, make the white sauce by mixing the Greek yoghurt, eggs, nutmeg, onion granules and garlic granules together in a bowl.

When the pasta is cooked, drain it and split in half. Take the saucepan with the mince off the heat. Pour one half of the pasta into the saucepan and add the passata and the tomato puree. Pour the other half of the pasta into the white sauce and stir.

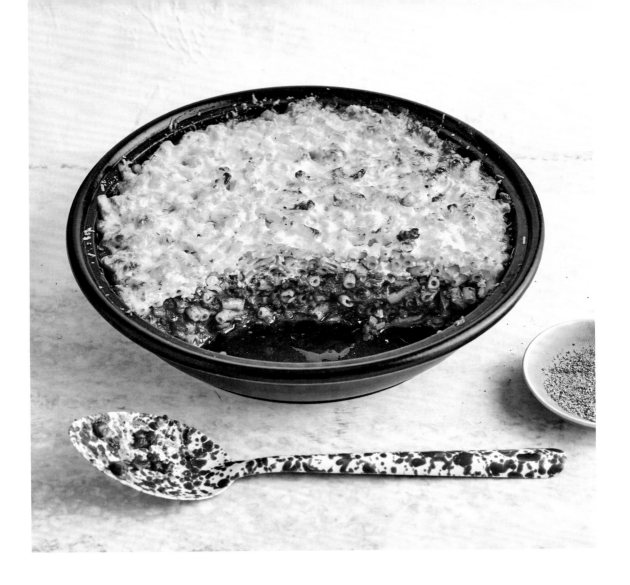

60g reduced-fat Cheddar
15g Parmesan

Spoon the pasta and the meat sauce mix into the bottom of a baking dish and spread it out. Spoon the pasta and white sauce mix on top of the meat sauce in the roasting dish. Grate the cheeses and scatter over the top.

Place the dish in the oven for 25 minutes, until the top is golden. Serve. The recipe can also be frozen once cooled – defrost fully then reheat until piping hot.

MAKE *it* VEGGIE

You can substitute the beef for 2 x 400g tins of green lentils, drained, and use a vegetable stock cube and Henderson's relish.

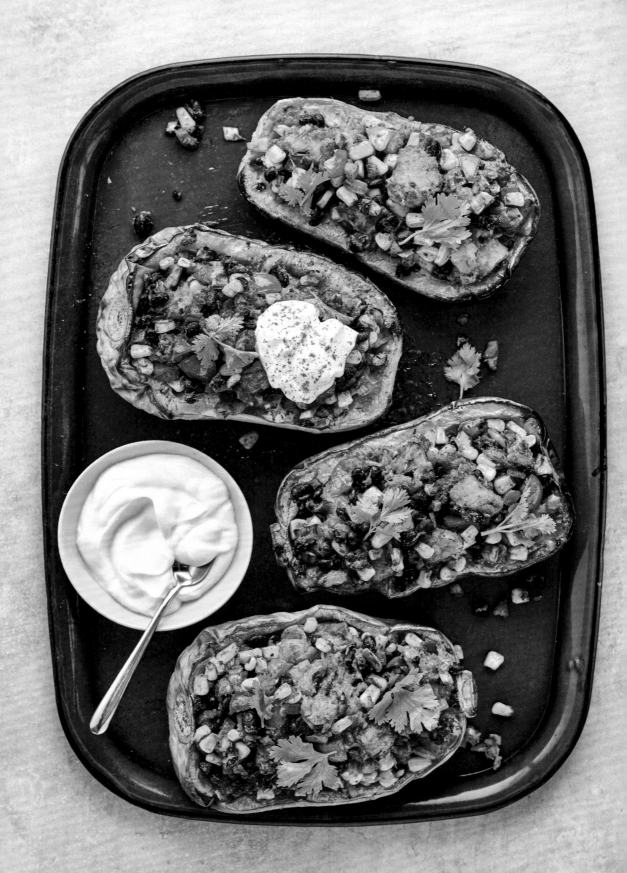

STUFFED SQUASH

🕐 **5 MINS** | 🍲 **60 MINS** | ✕ **SERVES 4**

This recipe is inspired by the amazing Mexican flavours of a burrito, but without all the heavy extras like rice and sour cream. Butternut squash is a great alternative to tortillas, and it is a great source of vitamin E and fibre – filling, nutritious and delicious. Perfect.

PER SERVING:
339 KCAL
48G CARBS

2 butternut squash, deseeded and cut in half lengthways (total 1.5kg)
low-calorie cooking spray
sea salt and freshly ground black pepper
2 white onions, peeled and finely chopped
1 x 400g tin black beans, drained
1 x 200g tin sweetcorn, drained
2 tomatoes, finely diced
2 tsp smoked paprika
2 tsp garlic granules
1 tsp ground cumin
4 tbsp Greek yoghurt
fresh coriander, to serve (optional)

TO ACCOMPANY *(optional)*
75g mixed side salad (+ 15 kcal per serving)

Preheat the oven to 220°C (fan 200°C/gas mark 7).

Spray the butternut squash all over with low-calorie cooking spray and season with salt and pepper. Place onto a baking tray and into the middle of the oven for 45 minutes, until they are cooked and you can push a fork into the flesh easily.

While the squash is cooking, gently sauté the onions in a frying pan with some low-calorie cooking spray. Cook over a medium heat for 5 minutes until softened, then set aside.

Once the squash is done, remove from the oven and let it cool while you prepare the stuffing. Mix the cooked onions in a bowl with the beans, sweetcorn, tomatoes, paprika, garlic, cumin and some salt and pepper.

Scoop the flesh out of the squash, roughly chop it and mix it with the beans. Spoon the mixture back into the skins and put them back into the oven for another 15 minutes.

When they are cooked, serve with a dollop of fat-free Greek yoghurt and fresh coriander, if desired. The recipe can also be frozen once cooled – defrost fully then reheat until piping hot.

Tip
This dish is also delicious with a little grated vegetarian hard cheese melted on top.

WELSH RAREBIT POTATOES

🕐 **5 MINS** | 🍲 **17 MINS** | ✕ **SERVES 2**

Who says baked potatoes need to be boring? These cheesy Welsh rarebit potatoes are the ultimate comfort food. Perfect for lunch or a light dinner, these are best served with a side salad to keep the calories low. Try experimenting with different toppings! Ham also works well.

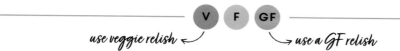

use veggie relish ↲   ↳ *use a GF relish*

PER SERVING:
307 KCAL
40G CARBS

2 baking potatoes (about 200g each), scrubbed
2 tsp Worcestershire sauce or Henderson's relish
1 tsp mustard powder
½ tsp garlic granules
75g light spreadable or squeezy cheese
sea salt and freshly ground black pepper
4 spring onions, trimmed and both green and white thinly sliced
low-calorie cooking spray
40g reduced-fat Cheddar, finely grated

TO ACCOMPANY *(optional)*
75g mixed side salad
(+ 15 kcal per serving)

Preheat the oven to 220°C (fan 200°C/gas mark 7).

Stab the potatoes with a fork, then microwave on high for 7 minutes. They should be firm but cooked; the skin will look a little wrinkled when they are ready. (You can also bake the potatoes in the preheated oven for about 45 minutes until they are soft in the middle when pricked with a fork.)

Remove the potatoes from the microwave and leave to cool for a few minutes until you can handle them comfortably. Slice the potatoes in half and scoop out the flesh, leaving the skin intact. Mash the potato flesh in a bowl with a fork, then add 1 teaspoon of the Worcestershire sauce, the mustard powder, garlic granules, spreadable cheese and salt and pepper to taste. Mix until combined and then stir in the spring onions.

Spray the outside of the potato skins with low-calorie cooking spray. Place on a baking tray and then scoop the mixture back into the potato skins. Sprinkle the Cheddar on the top of the potatoes and drizzle the other teaspoon of Worcestershire sauce on top. Place in the middle of the hot oven for 10 minutes.

When the cheese is bubbling remove from the oven and serve. (Or the potatoes can be cooled and put in the freezer to keep for another day.)

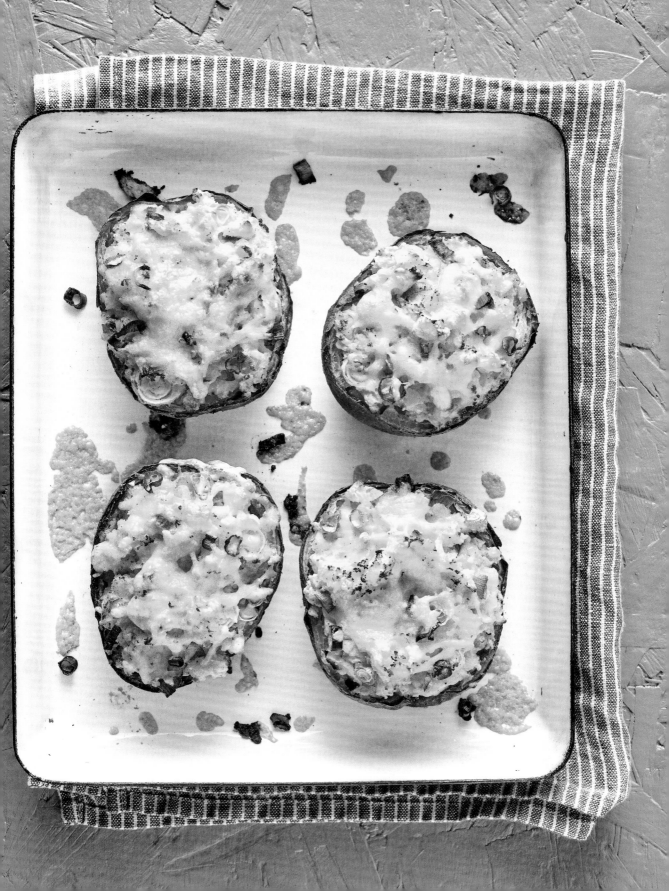

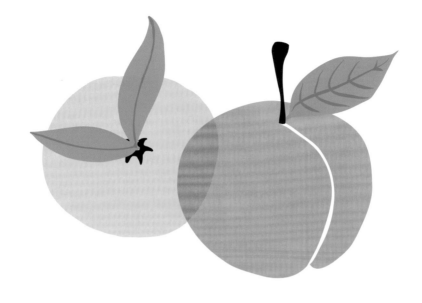

SNACKS, SIDES AND Sweet treats

BARBECUE POTATO WEDGES

⏱ **5 MINS** | 🍲 **45 MINS** | ✕ **SERVES 4**

Sometimes, you can't beat a classic side like barbecue wedges. Often found at a greasy takeaway, this version uses fresh ingredients and spicing from scratch, baked with a little low-calorie cooking spray, so you get the same smoky, delicious taste minus all the grease and calories. You can also freeze them for another day. Winner!

PER SERVING:
141 KCAL
29G CARBS

2 tsp all-purpose seasoning
1 tsp smoky paprika
1 tsp garlic granules
1 tsp onion granules
½ tsp celery salt
1 tsp dried oregano
pinch of dried chilli flakes, to taste
1 tsp granulated sweetener
sea salt and freshly ground
    black pepper
4 baking potatoes (about
    170g each), scrubbed
low-calorie cooking spray

Preheat the oven to 180°C (fan 160°C/gas mark 4) and line a baking tray with baking parchment.

In a small bowl, mix all of the herbs and spices, and the sweetener, together with a pinch each of salt and pepper. Cut each baking potato into wedges of around 1.5cm (½in) at the widest part, place in a large bowl and spray with low-calorie cooking spray. Sprinkle over the spice mix and toss until the wedges are well coated.

Place the wedges on the baking tray and spray with low-calorie cooking spray once more. Place in the oven for 45 minutes, turning them halfway through the cooking time. Serve while hot. The wedges can also be frozen once cooled – defrost fully before reheating.

Tip
These are a great accompaniment to our Quesadilla (see page 92).

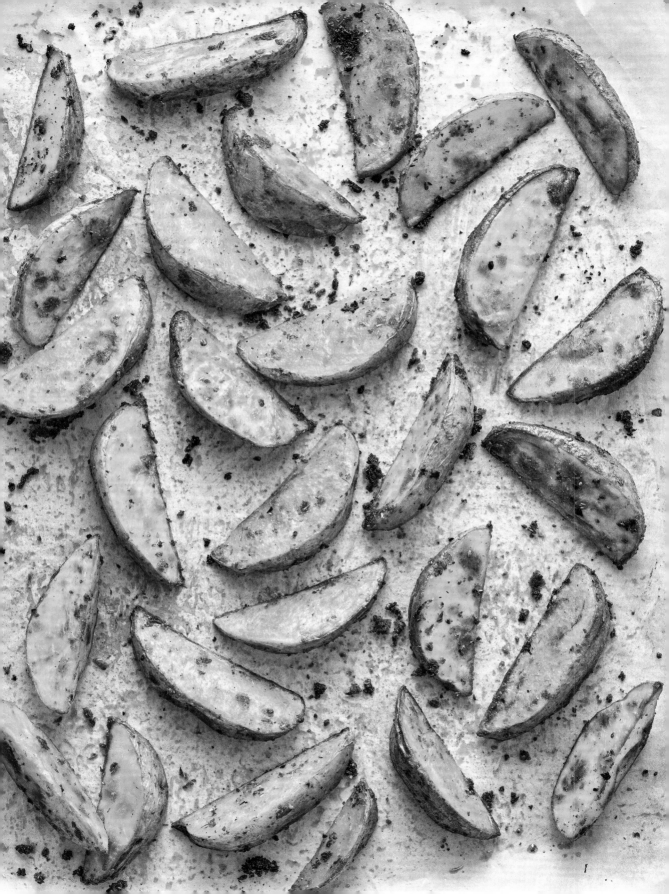

KATSU CHICKEN
SCOTCH EGGS

🕐 **15 MINS** | 🍲 **45 MINS** | ✕ **SERVES 2**

These Scotch eggs still taste like the real deal even though they are just 259 calories each. They are a match made in heaven served with katsu dipping sauce. Take them with you on your next picnic and impress your friends. Add a decent side salad to make this a hearty meal in itself.

PER SERVING:
259 KCAL
17G CARBS

2 medium eggs
3 large chicken sausages or
   4–6 chipolata-style sausages
½ tsp curry powder

FOR THE CURRY SAUCE
50g peeled potato, diced
55g peeled carrot, diced
55g peeled onion, diced
2 tsp curry powder
1 garlic clove, peeled and chopped
½ chicken stock cube
1 tsp tomato puree
300ml water

Preheat the oven to 200°C (fan 180°C/gas mark 6).

Place all of the ingredients for the sauce in a saucepan, bring to the boil, reduce the heat and simmer until the veg is cooked. This should take around 30 minutes or so.

While the sauce is cooking, place the eggs in a pan of boiling water and simmer for 6 minutes. When they are cooked, take them out and put them in a bowl of iced water. Leave to cool.

Remove the skins from the sausages and place the sausage meat in a bowl. Add the ½ teaspoon of curry powder and mix well. Set aside.

Peel the eggs carefully. Wet your hands to prevent the mixture sticking to your fingers, then use your hands to enclose an egg in half of the sausage meat, making a smooth ball. Repeat with the other egg, place them on a baking tray and cook in the oven for 15 minutes.

Once the veg for the sauce has cooked through, use a stick blender to blitz the contents of the saucepan until the sauce is smooth. If it's a little thick, you can add some more water until it reaches the desired consistency. Serve the eggs and sauce hot or cold. The sauce can be frozen once cooled – defrost fully before reheat or serving cold.

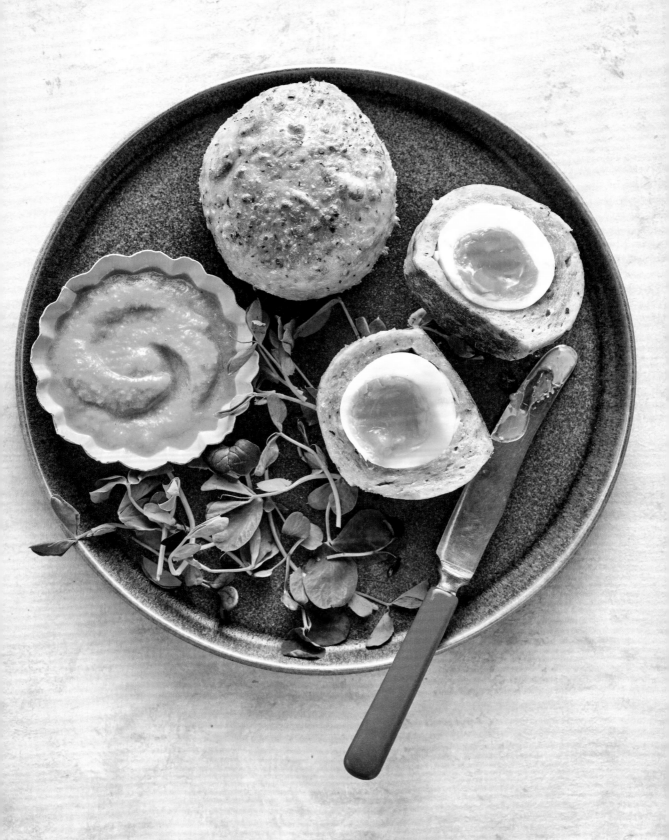

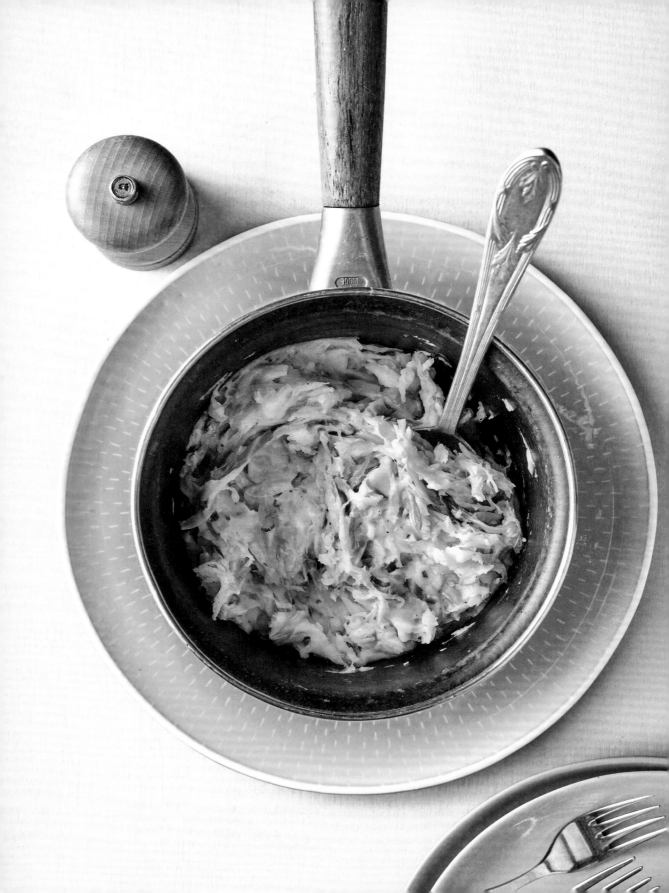

COLCANNON

⏱ **10 MINS** | 🍲 **20–25 MINS** | ✕ **SERVES 4**

This is such a simple recipe, but we promise that this Irish classic will change the way you view the lowly mashed potato. You can serve it as a side with roast meat, use it as a topping for a shepherd's pie, or however you would usually enjoy mash. It's so versatile. If you have leftovers, you can even fry it with low-calorie cooking spray and pop a fried egg on top for a tasty breakfast.

 V **F** **GF**

PER SERVING:
126 KCAL
25G CARBS

500g potatoes, peeled and cut into chunks
low-calorie cooking spray
200g savoy or green cabbage, finely shredded
4 spring onions, trimmed and thinly sliced
sea salt and freshly ground black pepper

Place the potato in a pan of boiling salted water. Bring back to the boil, turn the heat down and simmer until the potatoes are soft. This should take around 20–25 minutes.

While the potatoes are cooking, spray a frying pan with some low-calorie cooking spray, add the cabbage and spring onions and cook over a high heat until they are cooked, then set aside. This should take around 4 or 5 minutes.

When the potatoes are cooked, drain them well and return them to the pan, then, using a potato masher (or a stick blender with a masher attachment, if it has one), mash the potato until very smooth.

Stir in the cooked cabbage and spring onion, check the seasoning and add some salt and pepper if necessary, and serve. The colcannon can be frozen once cooled – defrost fully then reheat until piping hot.

Tip

Most modern stick blenders come with a masher attachment. We love them for making really smooth, silky mash.

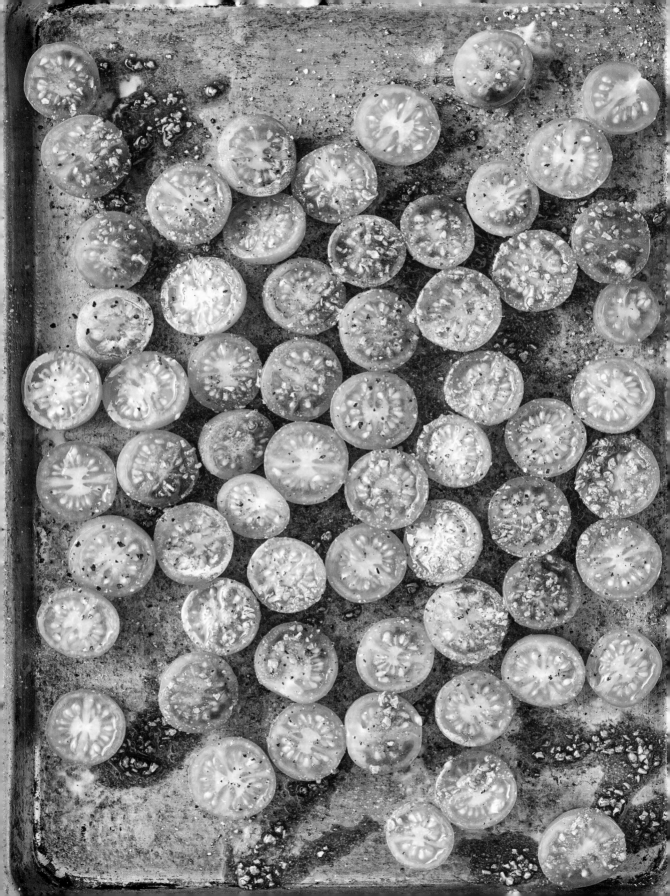

KETCHUP TOMATOES

🕐 **2 MINS** | 🍲 **20 MINS** | ✕ **SERVES 4**

These Ketchup Tomatoes are the perfect accompaniment to a cooked breakfast. Don't be put off if you normally avoid tomatoes with your full English – these are roasted, rich and sweet, just like your usual big splodge of ketchup.

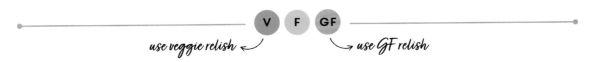

use veggie relish ↙   ↘ *use GF relish*

PER SERVING:
38 KCAL
4.7G CARBS

low-calorie cooking spray
350g cherry tomatoes,
   sliced in half
1 tbsp balsamic vinegar
1 tsp Worcestershire sauce
   or Henderson's relish
½ tsp sweet paprika
½ tsp onion granules
½ tsp garlic granules
sea salt and freshly ground
   black pepper

TO ACCOMPANY *(optional)*
Glamorgan Sausages, page 34
   and Cauliflower Tots, page 229
   (+ 322 kcal per serving)

Preheat the oven to 220°C (fan 200°C/gas mark 7).

Spray a baking tray with low-calorie cooking spray. Lay the cherry tomatoes, sliced side up, in one layer across the baking tray. Drizzle over the balsamic vinegar and Worcestershire sauce. Sprinkle over the paprika, onion granules and garlic granules. Season with salt and pepper. Spray with a little more low-calorie cookie spray and place in the middle of the hot oven.

After 20 minutes, when the tomatoes look roasted and dried out on top, remove from the oven and serve. The tomatoes can be frozen once allowed to cool.

Tip

Ketchup Tomatoes are not just for breakfast; you can cook up a batch of these and let them cool to use in salads and sandwiches.

MAC and CHEESE BITES

🕐 **15 MINS** | 🍲 **12 MINS** | ✕ **MAKES 24**

Macaroni cheese is the ultimate comfort food, but unfortunately not generally slimming-friendly! These mac and cheese bites hit the spot, without the added calories. Using strong cheese mixed with Cheddar means you get that classic cheesy taste without needing to use bags of the stuff. They are great for snacking, take no time to make, and are super cheesy – yum!

V **F**

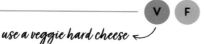
use a veggie hard cheese ↩

PER BITE:
38 KCAL
4.3G CARBS

low-calorie cooking spray
125g macaroni
1½ tsp chives, dried or
    freshly chopped
75g low-fat spreadable cheese
20g reduced-fat Cheddar, grated
pinch of mustard powder
sea salt and freshly ground
    black pepper
1 large egg, beaten
15g Parmesan or Italian hard
    cheese, grated

Preheat the oven to 190°C (fan 170°C/gas mark 5) and spray a 24-hole mini muffin tray with some low-calorie cooking spray.

Cook the macaroni according to the packet instructions, then drain and rinse in some cold water to stop it sticking together. Place the drained pasta in a bowl and stir in the chives, spreadable cheese, grated Cheddar and mustard powder. Season with some salt and pepper, mix well and check the seasoning. Stir in the beaten egg.

Divide the mixture equally between the twenty-four mini muffin moulds. Sprinkle the Parmesan over the top of each one and cook for 10–12 minutes, until they have set and browned on top.

Allow to cool for a minute or two before removing them from the muffin tray. Serve either warm or cold. The bites can also be frozen once cooled – defrost fully then reheat until piping hot.

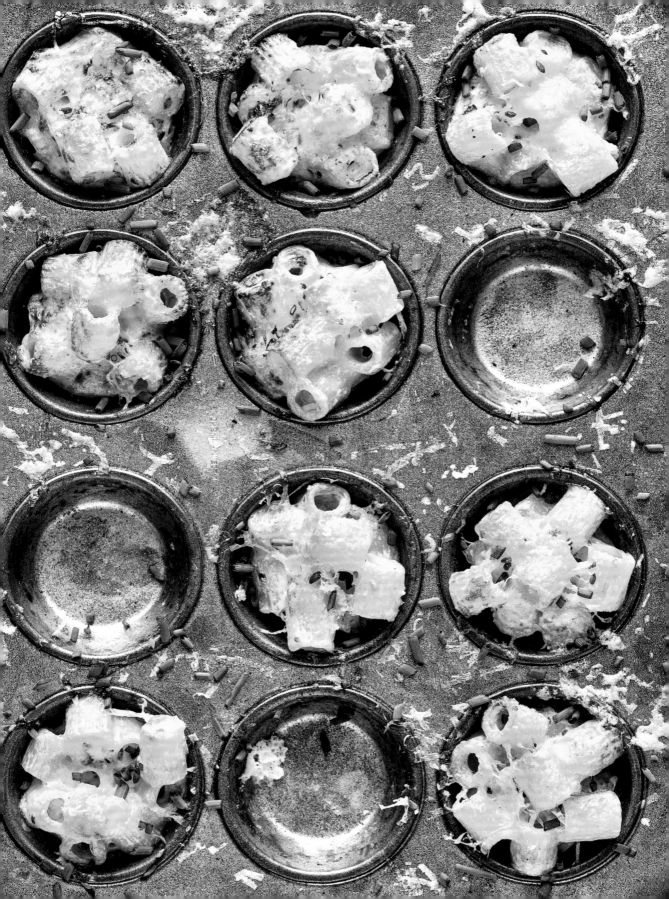

CORONATION POTATO SALAD

⏱ **5 MINS** | 🍲 **NO COOK** | 🍴 **SERVES 4**

There are two things that we love more than life itself: coronation chicken and potato salad. So the decision to make Coronation Potato Salad was like the accumulation of all life's loves in one. Creamy, mildly spiced potatoes with crispy spring onions and celery to add some crunch? Heaven. Literal heaven.

PER SERVING:
197 KCAL
40G CARBS

2 x 800g tins peeled new potatoes
120g fat-free natural yoghurt
1 tsp mild curry powder
½ tsp ground turmeric
½ tsp garam masala
1 tsp ground coriander
1 tsp granulated sweetener
1 celery stick, thinly sliced
6 spring onions, trimmed and
   thinly sliced
handful of chopped spinach leaves
sea salt and freshly ground
   black pepper
handful of fresh coriander leaves
   to serve (optional)

Drain the tins of potatoes and set to one side. Put the yoghurt, curry powder, turmeric, garam masala, ground coriander and sweetener in a bowl and mix. Add the potatoes, celery, spring onions and spinach to the bowl and mix together.

Season with salt and pepper and serve with fresh coriander sprinkled on top, if desired.

Tips

We've made this speedy by using tinned potatoes, but feel free to cook your own potatoes if you wish. You could also add 120g of chopped dried apricots for an extra 56 kcals per serving.

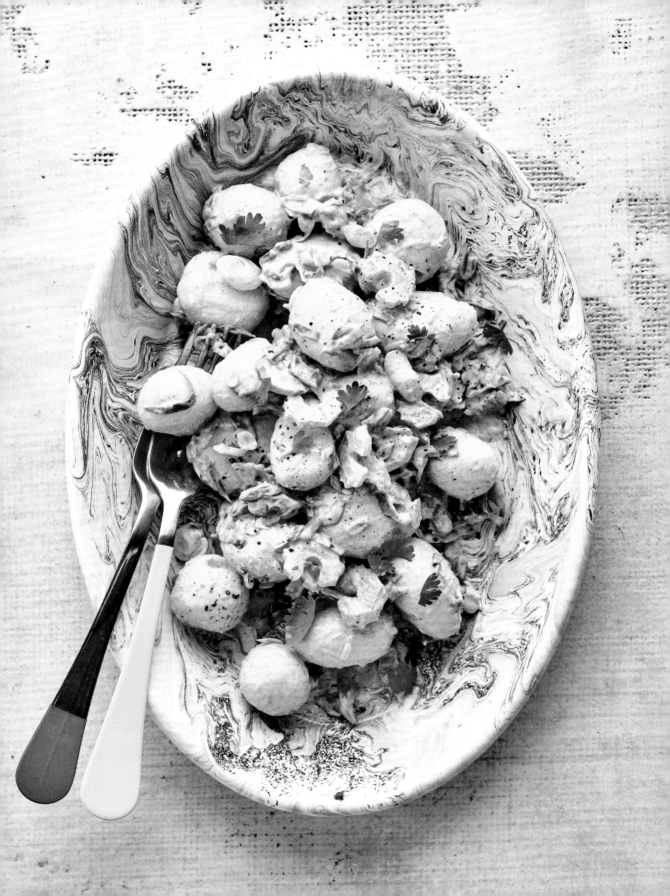

FRENCH PEAS

🕐 **5 MINS** | 🍲 **20 MINS** | ✕ **SERVES 4**

This recipe is based on the classic French dish Petits pois à la Français but don't be put off by the fancy name. These are really just pimped-up peas which taste soooo good and can be served with any lean meat or fish, our Coq au Vin (see page 161) or even on their own as a light lunch.

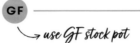

GF

→ use GF stock pot

PER SERVING:
108 KCAL
7.3G CARBS

low-calorie cooking spray
4 bacon medallions, thinly sliced
1 small onion, peeled and
    finely diced
3 garlic cloves, peeled and
    crushed
200ml vegetable stock
    (1 vegetable stock pot dissolved
    in 200ml boiling water)
200g frozen petits pois

Spray a large frying pan with low-calorie cooking spray and cook the bacon and onion for 5 minutes over a medium heat until the onion is translucent. Add the crushed garlic, mix into the bacon and onion and cook for another minute or so.

Add the stock and reduce over a high heat for 10 minutes. Stir in the peas and cook for another 4 minutes until the peas are just tender. Serve.

MAKE *it* VEGGIE

Replace the bacon with quorn
bacon-style rashers or slices.

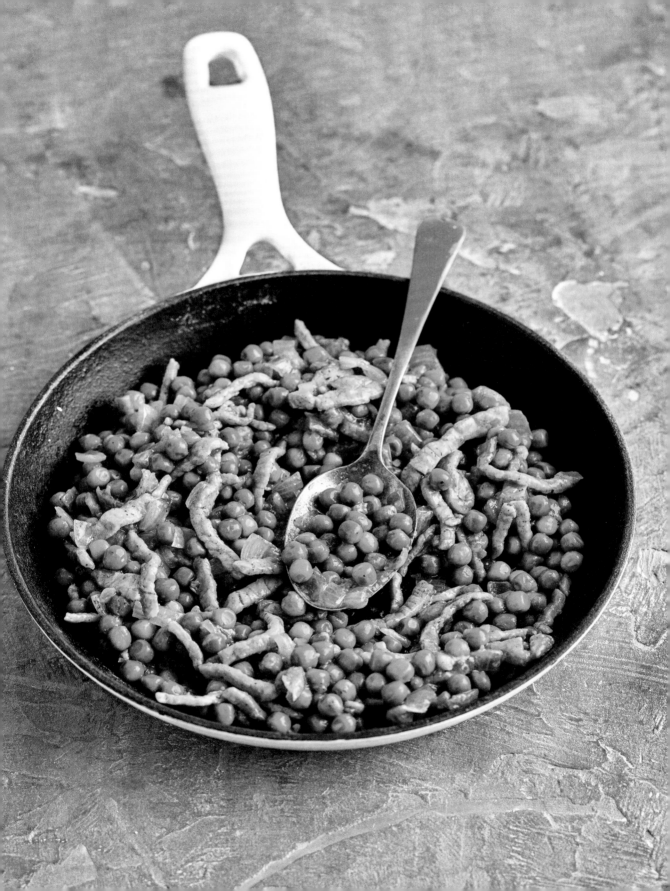

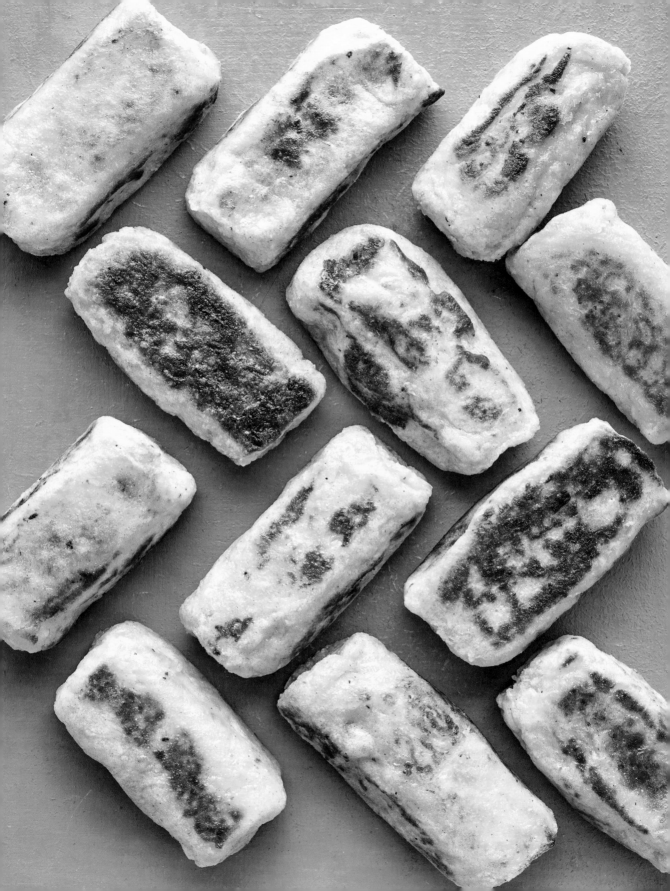

CAULIFLOWER TOTS

🕐 **5 MINS** | 🍲 **40 MINS** | ✗ **SERVES 4**

The potato counterparts of these are an American staple, but we have the perfect, healthier solution to those deep-fried versions. By adding cauliflower and baking instead of frying, these Tots have significantly fewer calories. Serve with Ketchup Tomatoes (see page 221) and Glamorgan Sausages (see page 34) for a full veggie breakfast at just 360 calories for the lot (1 sausage per portion)!

PER SERVING:
164 KCAL
22G CARBS

1 large potato, peeled and
   cut into 1cm (½in) cubes
   (about 240g)
1 head of cauliflower
   (about 600g), trimmed
1 tsp xanthan gum
1 tsp garlic granules
½ tsp onion granules
2 eggs, one for the mix, one
   beaten for basting
sea salt and freshly ground
   black pepper
low-calorie cooking spray

Preheat the oven to 220°C (fan 200°C/gas mark 7). Stab the potato with a fork, then microwave on high for 7–8 minutes until it is cooked. Remove from the microwave and allow to cool slightly. (Or, bake the potato in the oven for about 45 minutes until soft in the middle when pricked with a fork.)

Blitz the cauliflower in a food processor until it's the consistency of rice (you may need to do this in batches). Place in a bowl, cover with cling film and microwave for 10 minutes on high. It should be cooked but still have a firm texture. Allow to cool slightly, then use a clean tea towel or fine sieve to squeeze out excess moisture.

Halve the potato, scoop the flesh into a bowl, mash with a fork, then mix with the cauliflower, xanthan gum, garlic granules, onion granules and one of the eggs. Season with salt and pepper. The mixture will be sticky but hold together when you shape it.

Line a baking tray with foil and spray it liberally with low-calorie cooking spray. Shape the mix into 30–40 short sausage shapes, each around 2.5cm (1in) long, and place them on the baking tray, making sure there is room to turn them later. Baste the tops lightly with half of the second egg and spray with low-calorie cooking spray. Bake in the middle of the oven for 15 minutes.

Spray the tops of the tots with low-calorie cooking spray before very gently turning them. If they start to break apart, put them back in the oven for another 5 minutes before trying to turn them again. Baste with the rest of the egg, spray with low-calorie cooking spray and put back in the oven for 15 minutes until golden, crisp and hot in the middle. Remove from the oven and serve. The tots can also be frozen once cooled.

Tip

It's important to leave enough room on the tray to turn the tots. You have to be delicate, so spread them across two baking trays if you need to.

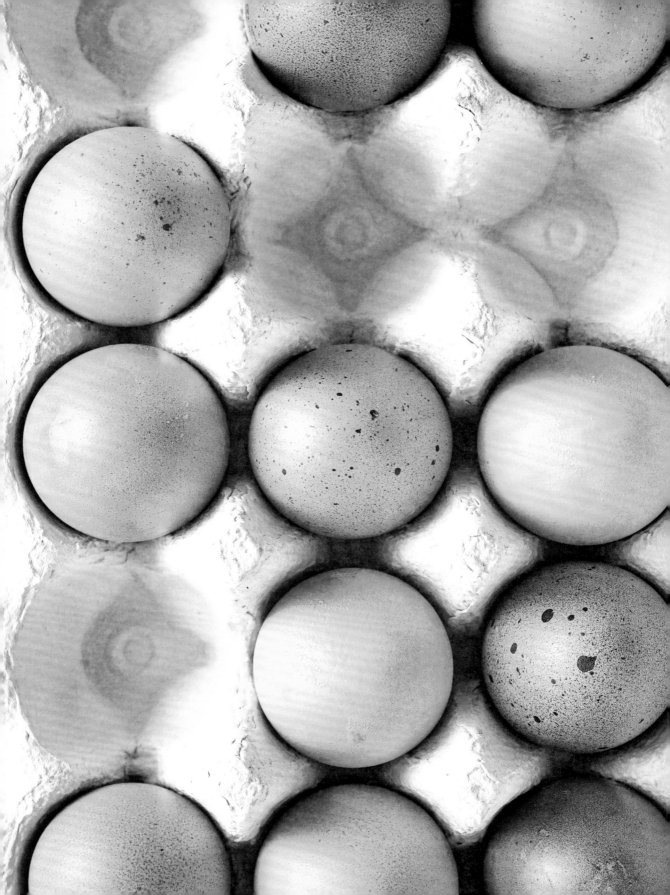

I MIGHT GET

ADDICTED

to the

GARLIC
SCALLOPED

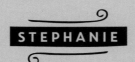

potatoes

— STEPHANIE —

The **KATSU SCOTCH EGGS** are surprisingly *easy* to make

CHELSEA

The **BARBECUE POTATO WEDGES** were *amazing*

MICHELLE

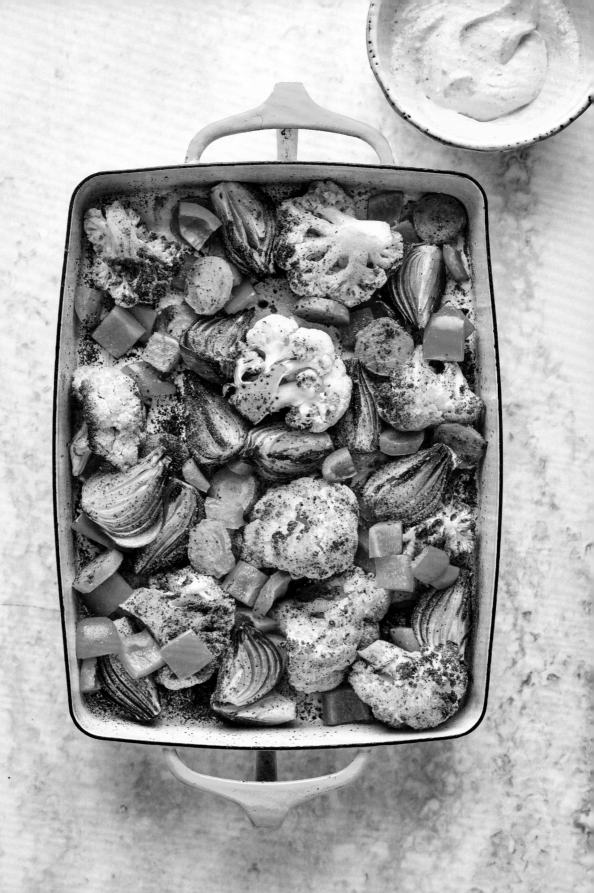

LOADED CAULIFLOWER TRAY BAKE

🕐 **5 MINS** | 🍲 **60 MINS** | ✕ **SERVES 6**

By roasting cauliflower in mild Indian spices and lemony sumac, we've elevated the humble vegetable into something much more special. Add the sweet yoghurt dressing and you'll find the dish becomes a new staple.

PER SERVING:
168 KCAL
28G CARBS

1 head of cauliflower, trimmed and split into evenly sized florets (600g)
6 red onions, peeled and sliced into quarters
3 carrots, peeled and chopped into 5mm (¼ in)-thick discs
low-calorie cooking spray
2 tsp ground turmeric
2 tsp sumac
2 tsp garlic granules
1 tsp onion granules
sea salt and freshly ground black pepper
2 red peppers, deseeded and diced

FOR THE DRESSING
150g fat-free Greek yoghurt
½ tsp garlic granules
½ tsp onion granules
½ tsp dried mint
½ tsp ground turmeric
½ tsp white wine vinegar
¼ tsp granulated sweetener
dash of water

Preheat the oven to 200°C (fan 180°C/gas mark 6).

Place the cauliflower, onions and carrots in a large roasting dish. Spray with low-calorie cooking spray until all the vegetables are coated. Sprinkle on the turmeric, sumac, garlic granules, onion granules and season with salt and pepper. Place the roasting dish into the middle of the oven for 40 minutes.

After 40 minutes, mix the veg up and coat with some more low-calorie cooking spray. Sprinkle the diced pepper on top and roast for a further 20 minutes. (At this point, you could allow the vegetables to cool, then freeze for another day.)

While the vegetables are finishing cooking, make the dressing. Mix together the yoghurt, garlic granules, onion granules, mint, turmeric, white wine vinegar and sweetener together in a bowl. Season with salt and pepper to taste and add a dash of water to thin the dressing.

When the vegetables are cooked through, remove from the oven, drizzle over the dressing and serve.

GARLIC SCALLOPED POTATOES

⏱ **5 MINS** | 🍲 **50 MINS** | ✕ **SERVES 4**

Kay often declared these crispy discs of potato a favourite as a child, referring to them as 'scallops', so that many people thought she had very refined taste for her age! They're a nice change from wedges or chips and, when seasoned with a little garlic and soft in the middle and crispy on the outside, we think you'll love them too. Serve with our Ratatouille Chicken recipe (see page 174) as an alternative to chips and potato wedges.

V F GF

PER SERVING:
176 KCAL
37G CARBS

800g potatoes, scrubbed
(skin left on)
low-calorie cooking spray
1 tbsp garlic granules
sea salt and freshly ground
black pepper

Preheat the oven to 220°C (fan 200°C/gas mark 7).

Slice the potatoes into 5mm (¼in)-thick discs (you don't need to peel them first). Place the potato slices in a microwavable dish and coat them with low-calorie cooking spray. Make sure all the slices are coated.

Microwave on high for 5 minutes. Shake the dish, making sure none of the slices are sticking together, and microwave on high for a further 5 minutes. The potatoes should be half cooked through, still firm and holding their shape. They will feel sticky from the starch. Sprinkle over the garlic granules and season with salt and pepper. Make sure the seasoning is evenly distributed over the slices.

Line a baking tray with foil or baking parchment and spray with low-calorie cooking spray. Lay the slices on top and spray with more low-calorie cooking spray. Place the tray into the middle of the hot oven for 25 minutes. When the potatoes look golden on top, flip them over, spray with a little more low-calorie cooking spray and put them back into the oven for another 15 minutes. When they are done, they should be crispy and lightly golden, like cooked potato wedges.

Remove from the oven and serve. The potatoes can also be frozen once cooled – defrost fully then reheat until piping hot.

Tip

These can also be cooked in an air fryer. Use the same method and timings for your model that you would use for chips (see page 48).

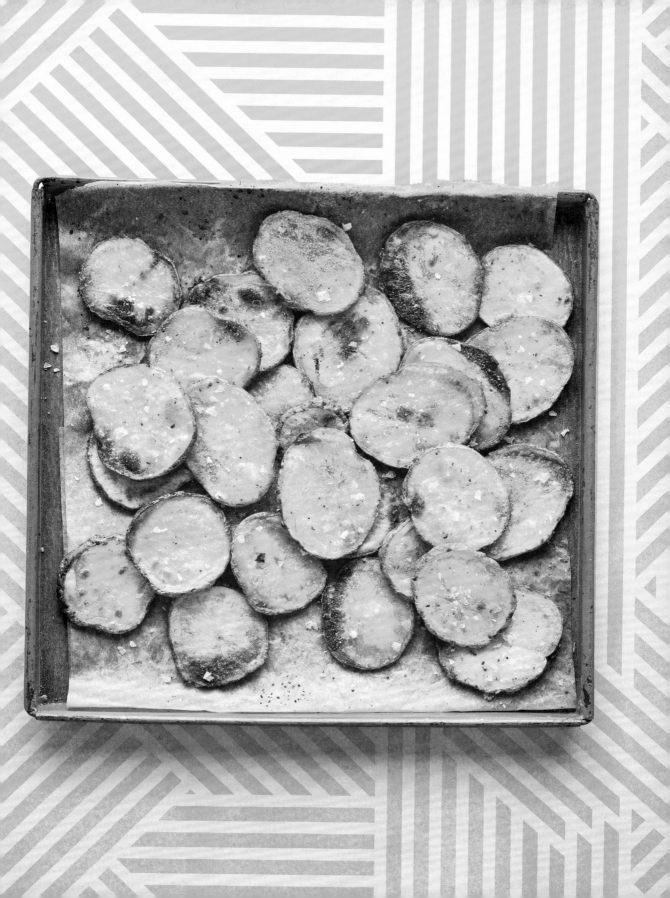

LEMON *and* CORIANDER HUMMUS

🕐 **2 MINS** | 🍲 **NO COOK** | ✗ **SERVES 4**

This hummus is fresh and zingy with lemon, making it the perfect dip for veggie sticks. We use butter beans to both reduce calories and give a creamier, less gritty texture than making it with chickpeas. This hummus goes well with salads, and the lemon flavour pairs well with grilled meats like chicken and fish, or our Seekh Kebab Roll (see page 53).

PER SERVING:
80 KCAL
13G CARBS

25g bunch of coriander,
  leaves only, plus extra leaves
  to serve
1 x 400g tin butter beans, drained
70g fat-free natural yoghurt
zest and juice of 1 lemon, plus
  extra slices to serve
2 tsp garlic granules
sea salt and freshly ground
  black pepper

Roughly chop the coriander leaves. Add half of the coriander to a blender with the butter beans, natural yoghurt, lemon juice and zest, garlic granules and a pinch each of salt and pepper. Blitz until coarsely blended, then stir in the other half of the coriander.

Serve, garnished with lemon slices and more coriander leaves.

Tip

Finely chop the stalks left over from your coriander bunch and pop them in the freezer. You can then add them to the pot next time you are cooking a curry or soup.

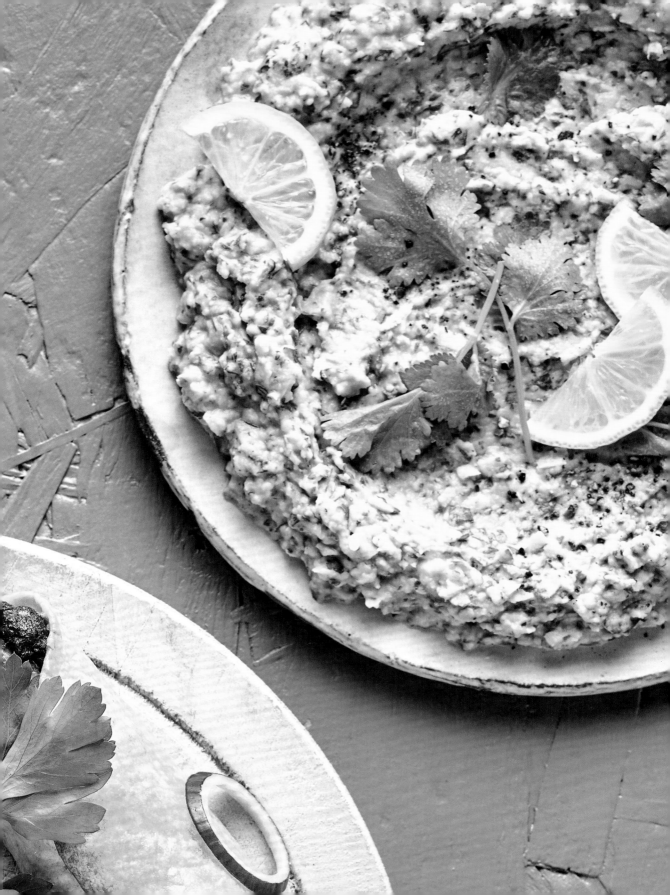

VEGETABLE
PARMESAN CHIPS

🕐 **5 MINS** | 🍲 **35 MINS** | ✕ **SERVES 2**

Having chips on the menu doesn't mean falling off the wagon. These crisp up really nicely in the oven and with the added rosemary and Parmesan, they taste incredible. Serve with yoghurt and a squeeze of lemon if you don't mind the extra calories.

use a veggie hard cheese ←

PER SERVING:
276 KCAL
28G CARBS

2 small carrots, peeled and trimmed
2 small parsnips, peeled and trimmed
1 small sweet potato, peeled about 120g
low-calorie cooking spray
60g Parmesan (or vegetarian hard cheese), finely grated
1 tbsp finely chopped fresh rosemary leaves
sea salt

Preheat the oven to 170°C (fan 150°C/gas mark 3).

Cut the carrots, parsnips and sweet potato into thin strips, about 5mm (¼ in) wide. Spread evenly onto a large baking tray lined with baking parchment and spray with low-calorie cooking spray.

In a small bowl, mix the finely grated Parmesan with the finely chopped fresh rosemary. You could use the same amount of dried rosemary too, but fresh is more fragrant and has a better flavour.

Sprinkle the cheese and herb mix over the chips and turn them to ensure an even coating. Place in the oven for 35 minutes or until golden. Check the chips after 25 minutes to make sure they're not beginning to burn on the edges.

Remove from the oven, sprinkle with salt as required and leave for 5 minutes before serving, as they will crisp up.

Tip

These can also be cooked in an air fryer. Use the same method and timings for your model that you would use for chips (see page 48).

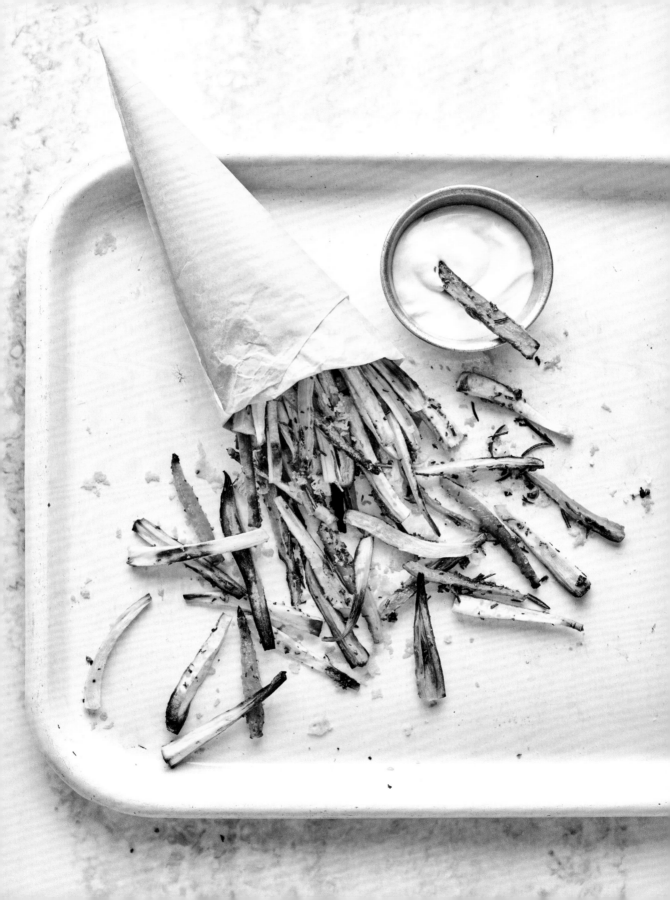

BROCCOLI CHEESE

🕐 **10 MINS** | 🗑 **15–20 MINS** | ✕ **SERVES 4**

This dish is often served as a side with a roast, but it absolutely stands alone as a quick, midweek meal that all of the family will love. Using stock alongside the cheese means the small amount of cheese goes much further, while still keeping the salty, cheesy, rich taste we all know and love. A touch of mustard lifts the cheese sauce to make it taste even cheesier – yum!

↘ *use a GF stock cube*

PER SERVING:
140 KCAL
9.2G CARBS

low-calorie cooking spray
½ onion, peeled and
    roughly chopped
1 garlic clove, peeled and chopped
250g cauliflower, trimmed
250ml vegetable stock
    (1 vegetable stock cube
    dissolved in 250ml
    boiling water)
½ tsp mustard powder
1 head of broccoli, trimmed
    (about 350g)
80g reduced-fat Cheddar
    cheese, grated
sea salt and freshly ground
    black pepper

Spray a saucepan with low-calorie cooking spray and sauté the onion and garlic over a low heat for around 3–4 minutes, until they have softened, but not browned. Cut the cauliflower into florets and place in a food processor. Blitz for a few seconds until fine. Place the cauliflower in the pan, then add the stock and mustard powder. Bring to the boil, then reduce the heat and simmer gently for 15 minutes.

Preheat the grill to high.

Cut the broccoli into florets and cook in a pan of boiling salted water for 5 minutes. Drain well and place in an ovenproof dish.

When the cauliflower is cooked, add three-quarters of the grated cheese and return the mix to the food processor. Blitz again, until you have a smooth sauce. Add a little water if it seems too thick. Season with salt and pepper to taste. (At this point the broccoli and cheese sauce can be frozen separately once cooled – defrost fully before using.)

Pour the cheese sauce over the broccoli and sprinkle on the remaining cheese. Place under the preheated grill, until the cheese has melted and is a golden brown.

Tip

Use a bag of cauliflower rice to reduce prep time.

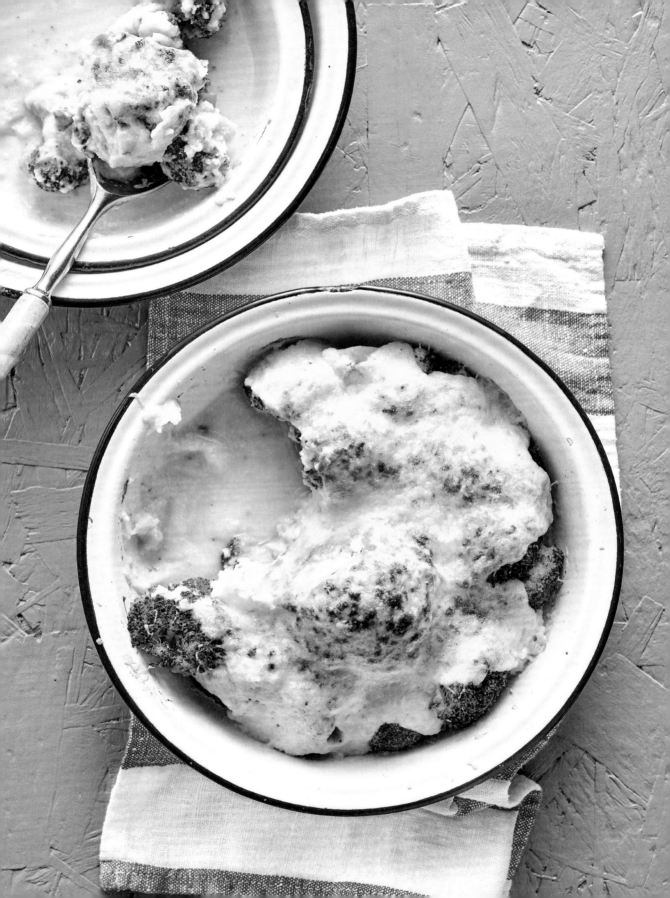

PINK APPLE SLAW

🕐 **10 MINS** | 🍲 **NO COOK** | ✕ **SERVES 4**

Sometimes it can be a struggle to find low-calorie meal accompaniments or sides, but by using some sharp and strong flavours such as lemon and cider vinegar, this slaw, heavy with juicy apple, is a real treat. So, so tasty and at just 40 calories per serving, it's an absolute winner with anything – we love it with our Popcorn Chicken recipe (see page 56).

PER SERVING:
40 KCAL
6.3G CARBS

2 tbsp cider vinegar
juice of ½ lemon
1 tbsp water
½ tsp granulated sweetener
½ tsp dried rosemary
1 pink lady apple, skin left on
 (about 113g)
½ red cabbage, finely shredded
5 spring onions, trimmed
 and sliced
sea salt and freshly ground
 black pepper

Mix the cider vinegar, lemon juice, water, sweetener and rosemary together in a large bowl.

Coarsely grate or cut the apple into thin strips (julienne). There is no need to peel it. Immediately, toss the grated apple in the vinegar and lemon juice mix. This will prevent the apple from going brown.

Add the cabbage and spring onions. Season with salt and pepper, mix well and serve.

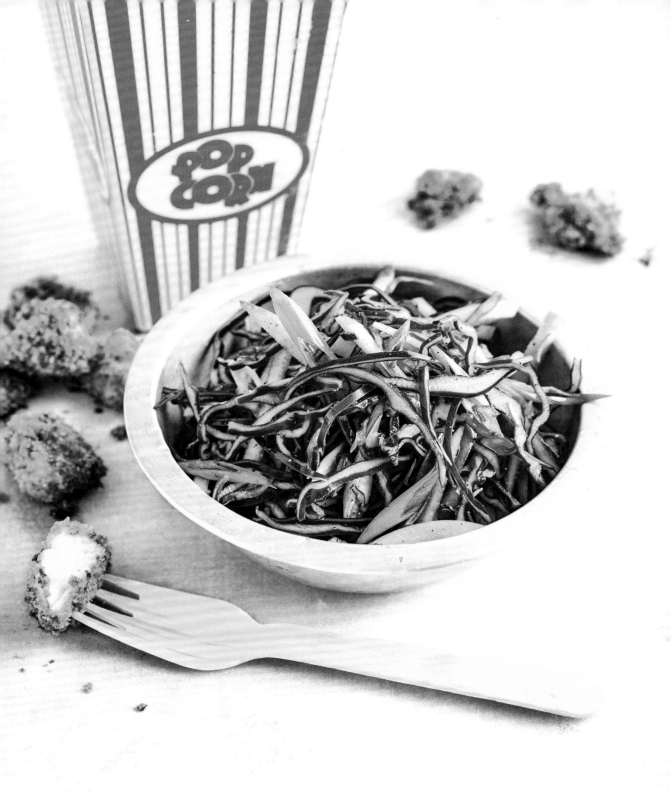

QUICKLES

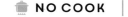 **10 MINS** (PLUS PICKLING TIME) | 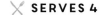 **NO COOK** | ✕ **SERVES 4**

Quickles (or quick pickles, if you're a party pooper) are great as a low-calorie snack, or to use in other recipes such as burgers or Sloppy Dogs (see page 65). We also love them served as part of our Ploughman's Platter (see page 95). Whereas regular pickles can take a week to ferment, these Quickles will be ready in a mere 40 minutes.

PER SERVING:
46 KCAL
5.8G CARBS

1 cucumber
2 tsp sea salt
200g radishes, sliced
1 medium red onion, peeled
　and sliced
3 tbsp white wine vinegar
2 tbsp granulated sweetener,
　or sugar if preferred

Cut the cucumber in half, then cut each half in half again lengthways. Using a teaspoon, scoop out the seeds and slice the cucumber.

Place the sliced cucumber in a colander and sprinkle with the salt. Cover with a plate and place an unopened tin on top (e.g. a tin of tomatoes or a tin of beans) to press out the excess water. Leave for 30 minutes, then remove the cucumber and pat it dry using some kitchen towel.

Place in a large bowl, add the remaining ingredients, stir well and serve.

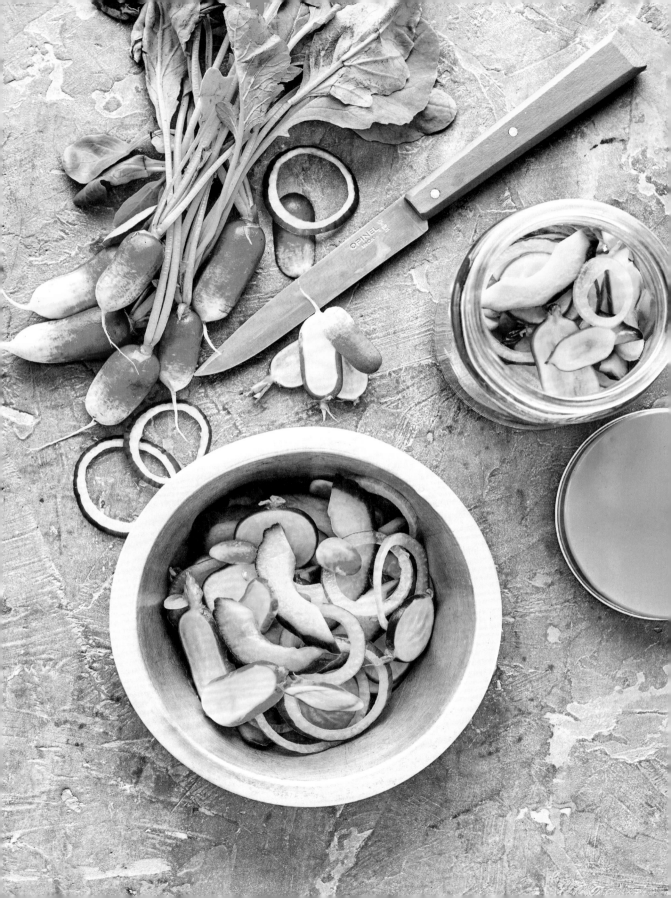

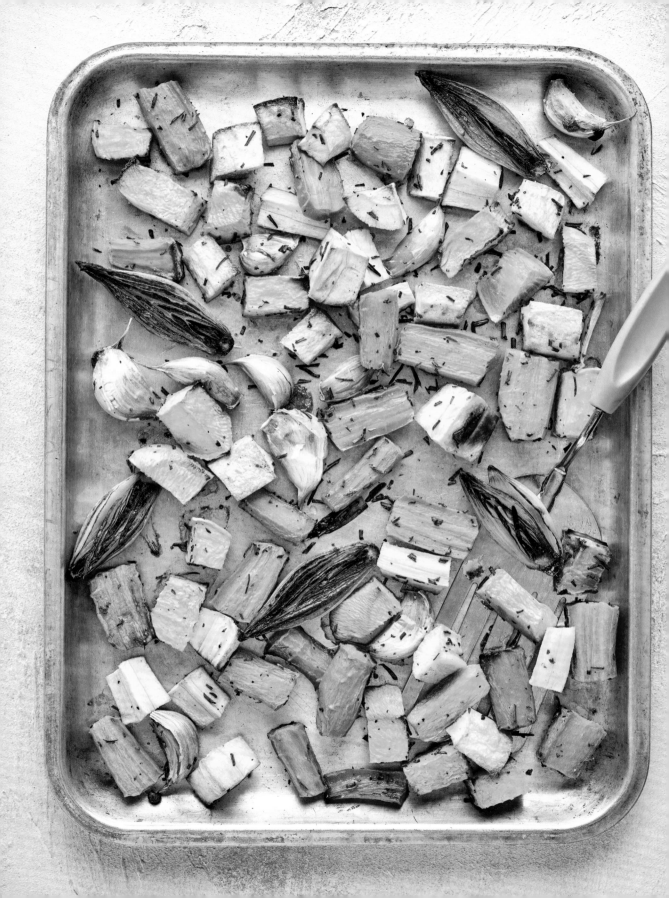

ROASTED ROOT VEGETABLES
with GARLIC *and* ROSEMARY

🕐 **10 MINS** | 🍲 **30-40 MINS** | ✗ **SERVES 4**

We are always looking for ways to get in our five a day, and these roasted veggies are way more appealing when mixed with garlic and rosemary. This flavour combination is a winner for Sunday lunch – we love it with our Herb-crusted Lamb recipe (see page 176). Fuss-free and simple, yet completely delicious!

PER SERVING:
140 KCAL
23G CARBS

1kg root vegetables (we used equal quantities of carrots, parsnips and swede)
1 garlic bulb
1 tbsp chopped rosemary
4 large shallots, peeled and cut into quarters
low-calorie cooking spray
sea salt and freshly ground black pepper

Preheat the oven to 180°C (fan 160°C/gas mark 4).

Peel the vegetables and cut into 2.5cm (1in) chunks. Peel the garlic cloves. Place the vegetables, garlic, rosemary and shallots in a large bowl. Spray with low-calorie cooking spray and season well with salt and freshly ground pepper.

Tip the vegetables onto a large baking tray and place in the oven. Cook for 15 minutes, then remove and gently turn the veg to ensure even cooking. Return to the oven for 15 more minutes, or until the vegetables are soft and golden brown. Remove from the oven and serve.

Tip
We always peel garlic cloves, but some cooks prefer to leave the skin on in the oven, then squeeze out the garlic flesh after roasting. The choice is yours!

RUSSIAN SALAD

🕐 **5 MINS** | 🍲 **20 MINS** | ✕ **SERVES 6**

This is a salad, but not as you know it! The vegetables are first cooked and then the dish is left to cool to room temperature before serving. Usually calorie-laden in mayonnaise, we've cut the calories using some perfectly balanced flavours and quark. It's a hearty side dish that's a little different.

PER SERVING:
119 KCAL
17G CARBS

360g carrots (about 5), peeled and
   cut into 1cm (½in) cubes
1 small swede, peeled and cut into
   1cm (½in) cubes
1 medium potato, peeled and cut
   into 1cm (½in) cubes (about 213g)
125g frozen peas
250g quark or fat-free
   natural yoghurt
½ tsp garlic granules
½ tsp dried dill
½ tsp mustard powder
10g fresh parsley, chopped
¼ tsp granulated sweetener
1 celery stick, finely chopped
6 cornichons or small gherkins,
   finely diced
1 tsp white wine vinegar
sea salt and freshly ground
   black pepper

In a large saucepan add the carrots, swede and potato, cover with cold water and bring to the boil. Once the water has reached boiling point, turn down to a simmer and put on the lid. Cook for 12 minutes.

Remove the lid and add the peas. Cook for a further 3 minutes until the peas are cooked. The swede, potato and carrots should be soft enough to pierce with a fork, but still firm enough to hold their shape. Drain the water from the pan and set the vegetables aside to cool.

While the vegetables are cooling, mix the quark, garlic, dill, mustard powder, parsley and sweetener to make the dressing.

Mix the cooled vegetables with the celery, cornichons, white wine vinegar and dressing. Season well with salt and pepper and serve.

Tip
A couple of chopped boiled eggs also make a great addition to this salad.

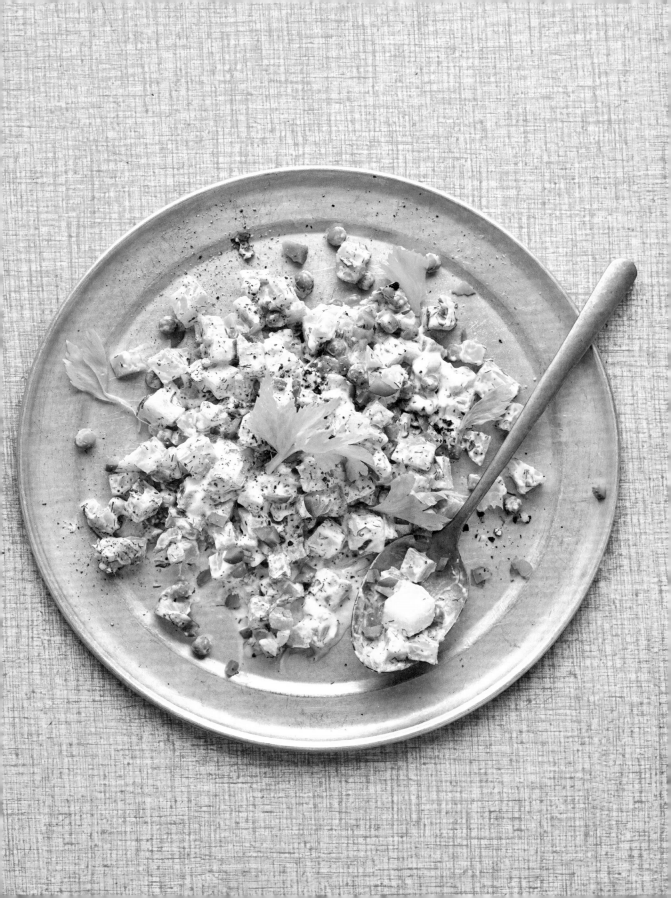

BATATAS PICANTES

⏱ **10 MINS** | 🍲 **60 MINS** | ✗ **SERVES 6**

We've given the classic patatas bravas the Pinch of Nom twist, and used sweet potatoes and low-fat cooking spray to keep the calories down. These are a perfect treat for dinner parties, where everybody can help themselves to everything they fancy. We used sweet paprika in this recipe, but feel free to use a hot one if you like it with a bit more spice.

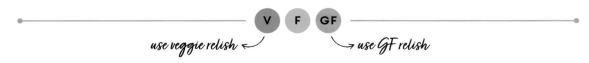

use veggie relish ↙   **V F GF**   ↘ *use GF relish*

PER SERVING:
220 KCAL
42G CARBS

1kg sweet potatoes, peeled
　and diced
low-calorie cooking spray
sea salt and freshly ground
　black pepper
1 tbsp sweet paprika
1 tbsp garlic granules
1 tbsp onion granules

FOR THE SAUCE
1 x 500g carton passata
2 tbsp balsamic vinegar
1 tbsp Worcestershire sauce
　or Henderson's relish
1 tsp sweet paprika
1 tsp garlic granules
½ tsp chilli powder
sea salt and freshly ground
　black pepper

Preheat the oven to 220°C (fan 180°C/gas mark 6).

Put the potatoes into a large roasting dish and spray liberally with low-calorie cooking spray. Season the potatoes with salt and pepper and the paprika, garlic granules and onion granules, making sure to toss them and coat them evenly. Spread them out so they are in a single layer. Put the roasting dish into the middle of the preheated oven for around 1 hour, making sure to turn occasionally.

Put the passata, balsamic vinegar, Worcestershire sauce, paprika, garlic granules, chilli powder and a pinch each of salt and pepper in a saucepan. Gently heat just before the potatoes are ready.

When the potatoes are done, they should be a little crispy and firm, like potato wedges. If they are not spread out in a single layer, they may take a little longer to cook. Once the potatoes are ready, remove from the oven. (At this point you can cool and freeze the potatoes for later, and do the same with the sauce, separately.)

Pour over the sauce and serve.

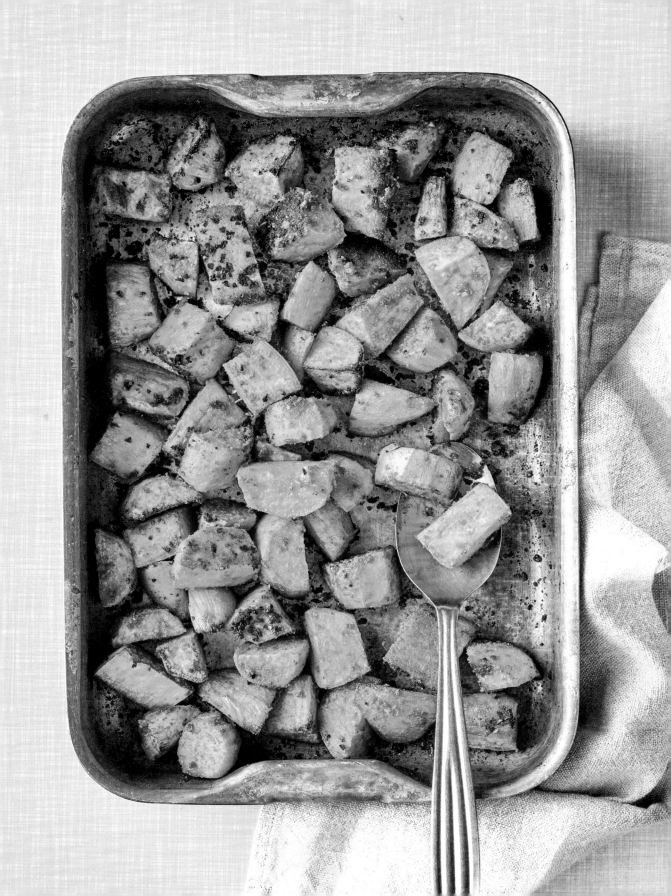

PEACHES *and* CREAM FRENCH TOAST

🕐 **5 MINS** | 🗑 **10 MINS** | ✗ **SERVES 4**

French toast is the ultimate luxurious dessert and, thankfully, you can still enjoy a lower-calorie version which tastes just as good. The peach adds a little sharpness to cut through the sweet flavour of the toast itself, while the creamy Greek yoghurt is rich and delicious. It is easy to halve or double this recipe.

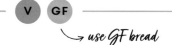

→ *use GF bread*

PER SERVING:
229 KCAL
19G CARBS

4 large eggs
4 tsp granulated sweetener
4 tsp vanilla extract
300g fat-free Greek yoghurt
4 tbsp no-added-sugar
   peach squash
low-calorie cooking spray
120g wholemeal bread, sliced
   (this will be around 4 slices;
   with or without crusts is fine)
2 peaches, stoned and sliced

In a bowl, whisk the eggs, sweetener and vanilla extract. In a second bowl, mix the yoghurt and peach squash.

Place a large frying pan on a low–medium heat and spray with low-calorie cooking spray.

Dip each slice of bread into the egg mixture, fully covering it with the egg and leaving it to soak in for 10 seconds per side. Put the egg-soaked bread straight from the egg into the frying pan and repeat for each slice.

Flip each slice after about 2 minutes, when it should be golden.

Once each side has cooked, assemble on a plate, spreading the peachy yoghurt onto the French toast and topping with slices of fresh peach.

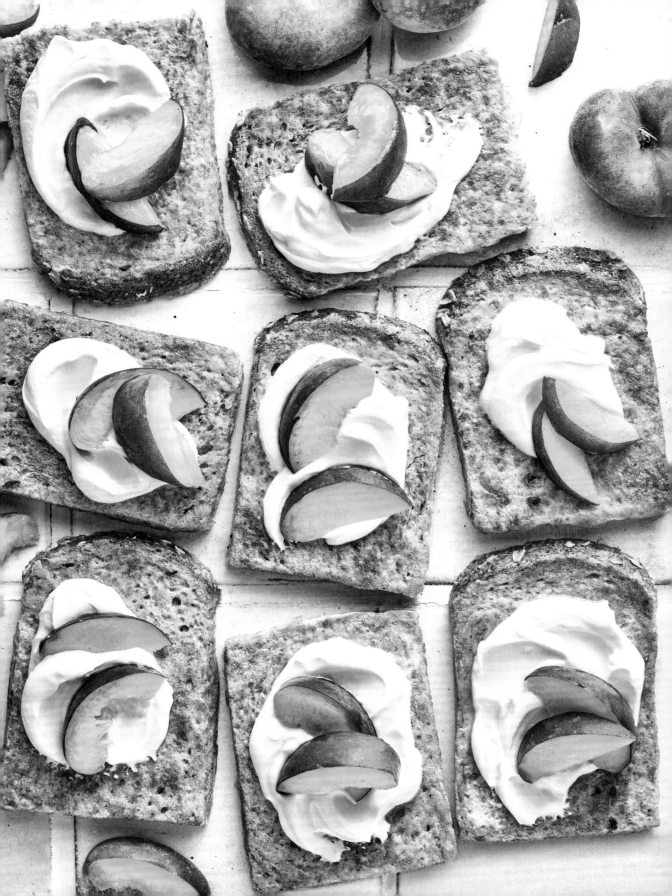

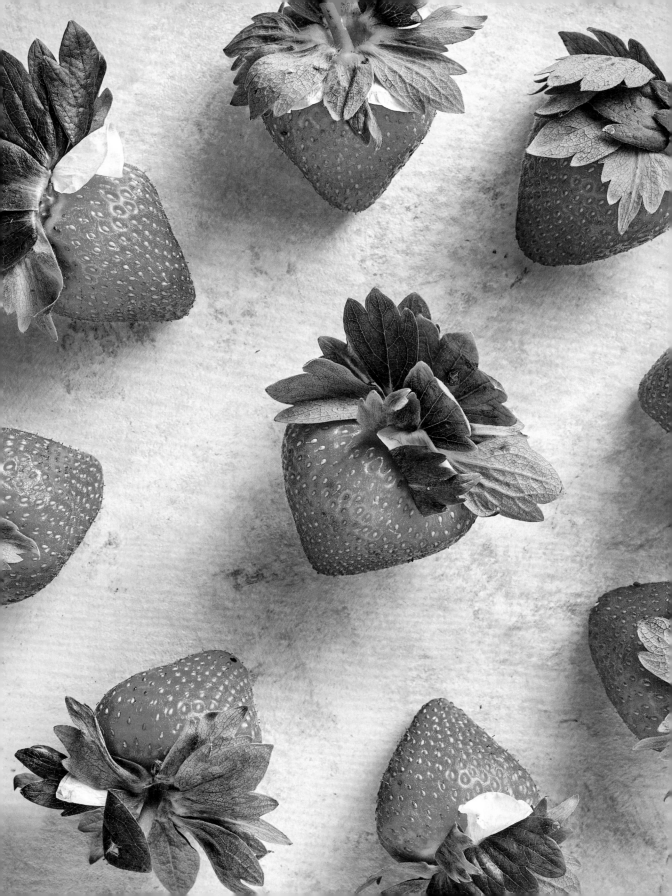

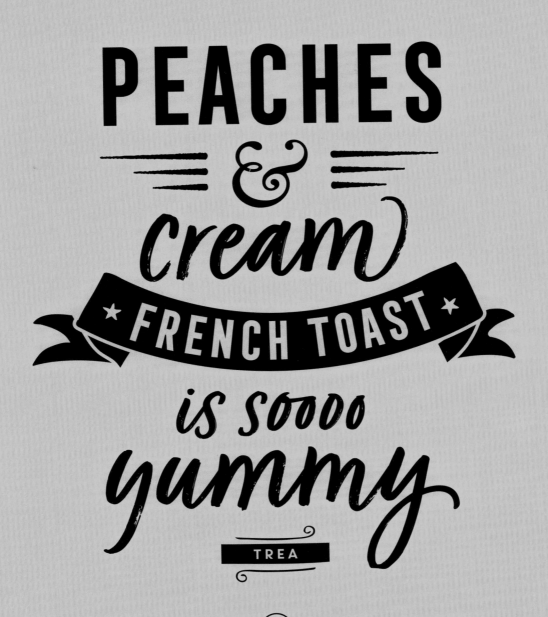

PEACHES

&

cream

FRENCH TOAST

is soooo

yummy

TREA

> RASPBERRY AND ELDERFLOWER SWIRL is a *great* alternative to ice cream. Super *creamy* and very *tasty*

HARRIET

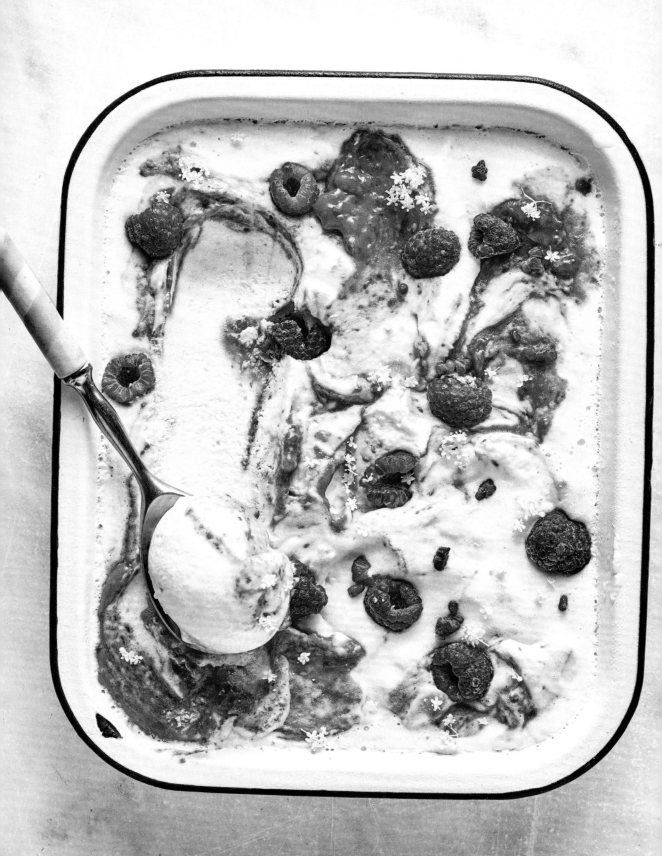

RASPBERRY *and* ELDERFLOWER SWIRL

🕐 **10 MINS** (PLUS FREEZING TIME) | 🍲 **NO COOK** | ✗ **SERVES 8**

If you're craving a creamy, ice cream dessert, then this is just the thing for you. Fat-free Greek yoghurt is naturally thick and makes a delicious alternative to ice cream when frozen. We've added some sharp raspberries and the sweetness of sugar-free elderflower cordial for an indulgent, tasty treat without all the calories of traditional ice cream!

PER SERVING:
114 KCAL
9.4G CARBS

1kg fat-free Greek yoghurt
80g granulated sweetener
4 tsp vanilla extract
200g fat-free natural yoghurt
350g frozen raspberries
200ml sugar-free elderflower cordial
1 tsp red food colouring

Place the yoghurt in a large freezable container and freeze for 4 hours.

Remove the frozen yoghurt from the freezer and place into a food processor or blender – you may need to scoop it out into large chunks in order to fit it in. Add the sweetener, vanilla extract and natural yoghurt and blend the yoghurt until smooth. Pour back into the freezable container.

In a bowl, mix the frozen raspberries with the elderflower cordial and red food colouring. Divide the raspberry mixture in half and set one half aside. Blitz the other half in your food processor or blender to form a paste. Stir this through the yoghurt lightly, to leave a ripple effect.

Place the reserved raspberry and elderflower mixture onto the top of the frozen yoghurt, pushing some of the raspberries into it by gently swirling a spoon through the mixture. Return to the freezer for a further 4 hours, or until ready to serve. Remove from the freezer and leave to thaw for around 10 minutes before scooping out.

STRAWBERRY *and* PEACH ICE LOLLIES

🕐 **5 MINS** (PLUS FREEZING TIME) | 🫕 **NO COOK** | ✕ **SERVES 8**

Shop-bought ice lollies can be laden with sugar and preservatives, so we made it our mission to create a fresh and healthy alternative. These Strawberry and Peach Ice Lollies are made with frozen strawberries which are so refreshing and sweet. Perfect for a summer afternoon.

PER SERVING:
9 KCAL
1.4G CARBS

150ml no-added-sugar
   peach squash
6 fresh or frozen strawberries
½ tsp red food colouring

Add 150ml water to a jug with the peach squash, keeping back 1 tablespoon of the undiluted peach squash. Mix well.

Chop the strawberries into quarters and place into the ice lolly moulds. Pour in the strong squash mixture. Depending on the size of your moulds, you may need more or less of the liquid – the ratio is 1 part water to 1 part squash.

Mix the food colouring in with 1 tablespoon of the neat squash. Drop a little into each lolly.

Assemble the moulds accordingly – either with sticks or lids, if making popsicles. Freeze for at least 4 hours, or preferably overnight. Release from the moulds by dipping in hot water for a few seconds and enjoy immediately!

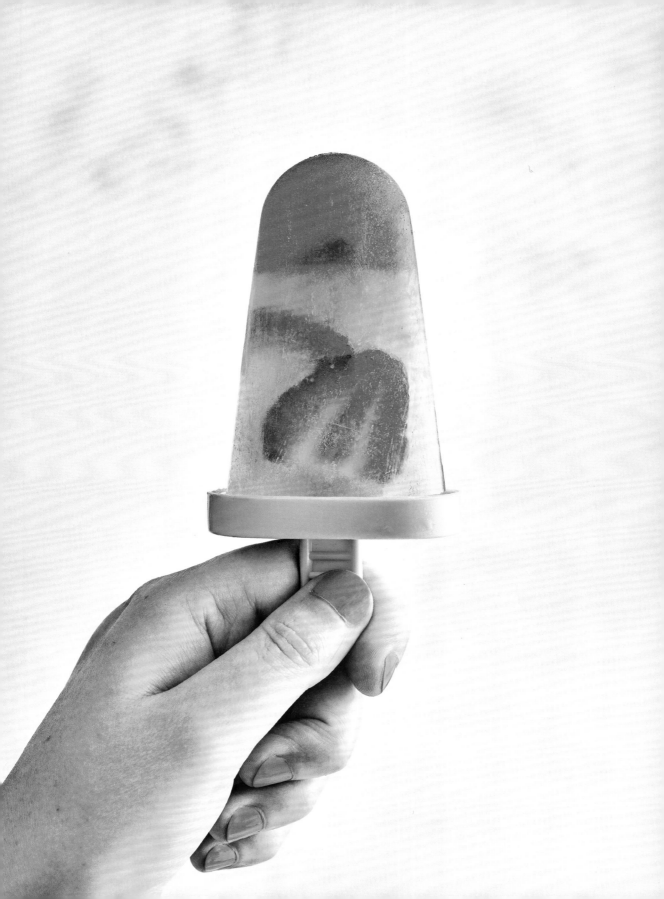

NUTRITIONAL INFO PER SERVING

Breakfast	ENERGY KJ/KCAL	FAT (G)	SATURATED FAT (G)	CARBS (G)	SUGAR (G)	FIBRE (G)	PROTEIN (G)
MONTE CRISTO SANDWICH	1591/379	15	5.3	28	4.1	5.5	29
BREAKFAST BANANA SPLIT	977/232	5.7	0.5	27	25	3.8	14
CHEESY LEEKS ON TOAST	1406/335	11	5.7	35	7.6	7.3	20
EGG-IN-THE-HOLE BREAKFAST BAGEL	1365/325	11	2.4	27	4.7	3	29
SAUSAGE & EGG ENGLISH MUFFIN	1586/377	12	4.5	26	4.9	4.4	38
GLAMORGAN SAUSAGES	662/158	7.3	3.3	13	1.3	1.5	9.8
GIANT BAKED BEANS	612/144	0.9	0.1	24	9.4	6.8	9.9
HASH BROWN BREAKFAST BAKE	797/189	2.7	0.5	23	5.4	5.1	16
ROSTI WAFFLE WITH ASPARAGUS & POACHED EGG	1182/281	7	1.8	38	3.2	6	13
HALLOUMI & SMOKY BACON HASH	1564/374	17	7.5	15	6.6	4.9	37

FAKEAWAYS	ENERGY KJ/KCAL	FAT (G)	SATURATED FAT (G)	CARBS (G)	SUGAR (G)	FIBRE (G)	PROTEIN (G)
CRYING TIGER BEEF	1529/362	6.7	2.3	12	9.3	3.1	60
FISH & CHIPS	1409/333	2.8	0.6	42	2.4	5.3	32
SEEKH KEBAB ROLLS	1234/293	6.6	2.5	25	3.6	4.5	31
CHICKEN TIKKA DRUMSTICKS	510/121	2.6	0.7	7.3	6.8	0.5	17
POPCORN CHICKEN	1500/356	7.1	1.7	24	1.8	4.9	46
CHIPOTLE PORK BURGER	1491/355	13	3	27	2.6	5.4	29
YEUNG CHOW FRIED RICE	1715/400	10	3.2	52	7.9	6.1	27
SLOPPY DOGS	1592/379	10	3.4	34	13	12	30
CHICKEN IN ORANGE	813/ 192	3	0.5	7.8	6.3	2.2	32
CRISPY CHINESE TURKEY WRAPS	1078/255	3.3	0.9	28	7.4	3.7	26

FAKEAWAYS Continued...	ENERGY KJ/KCAL	FAT (G)	SATURATED FAT (G)	CARBS (G)	SUGAR (G)	FIBRE (G)	PROTEIN (G)
GARLIC & LIME BALTI	952/223	2.5	0.5	18.8	16.4	6.9	31.7
FIRECRACKER PRAWNS	738/175	1.8	0.4	15	11	4.1	22
PIZZA-LOADED FRIES	1645/390	9	5.6	55	9.6	7.8	16

Quick MEALS	ENERGY KJ/KCAL	FAT (G)	SATURATED FAT (G)	CARBS (G)	SUGAR (G)	FIBRE (G)	PROTEIN (G)
ORANGE, CARROT & BEETROOT SALAD	265/63	0.5	0.1	11	11	3	1.4
MELT-IN-THE-MIDDLE FISHCAKES	1150/273	8.2	4.4	24	2.5	2.8	24
CAULIFLOWER-BASE PIZZA	1419/340	17	9.6	16	11	7.1	27
ASPARAGUS, BROAD BEAN & BACON SALAD	745/177	5.4	0.9	8.4	3.3	3.7	22
BROCCOLI, CHILLI & KING PRAWN STIR FRY	603/143	2.5	0.5	7.6	4.2	5.2	20
ASIAN PORK MEATBALLS	1142/272	9.3	1.3	12	9.1	3.1	32
CHICKEN & ASPARAGUS QUICHE	803/192	10	3.4	4.3	3.1	2.5	20
QUESADILLA	1061/252	5.2	3.3	32	7	7.1	15
PLOUGHMAN'S PLATTER WITH HOMEMADE CHUTNEY	1719/382	12.7	4.9	43.9	22.9	7	24.2
LEMON & PEPPER CHICKEN TAGLIATELLE	1680/397	6.6	1.8	35	1.3	2	48
HAM & POTATO CAKES	1091/259	5	1.4	33	2.7	3.9	18
SAUSAGE & ONION PLAITS	1130/268	6.6	1.1	27	5.6	3.5	23
SPINACH & RICOTTA STUFFED MUSHROOMS	309/74	4.2	1.8	3.9	2.8	1.4	4.5
MEDITERRANEAN VEGETABLE STUFFED MUSHROOMS	637/152	7.2	3.7	9.4	7.8	3.5	9.9
PORK, SAGE & ONION STUFFED MUSHROOMS	229/54	1.5	0.5	2.4	2.2	1.2	7.2
TANDOORI SALMON WITH MANGO SALSA	1483/355	19	3.4	13	12	3.6	32
THAI-SPICED FISH WITH NOODLES	1439/340	3	0.6	41	7	4.6	35
WARM GREEN BEAN AND FETA SALAD	465/111	4.5	2.6	6.9	5.1	3.3	8.9

BATCH COOK	ENERGY KJ/KCAL	FAT (G)	SATURATED FAT (G)	CARBS (G)	SUGAR (G)	FIBRE (G)	PROTEIN (G)
THAI CHICKEN CAKES	840/198	2.5	0.6	6	3.6	1.4	37
CHIPOTLE TURKEY MEATBALLS	1407/333	3.6	0.8	34	15	6	35
CHEESE & ONION CRISPBAKES	1262/300	9.5	3.9	36	2.5	5.4	15
HOT & SOUR SOUP	411/98	3.3	0.6	9	6.8	5.7	5
OVEN-BAKED RISOTTO WITH SMOKED SALMON & PEAS	1550/366	4.5	0.8	65	4.1	3.5	14
BUTTER BEAN & SWEET POTATO TIKKA MASALA	976/232	1.8	0.3	43	19	9	10
JAMBALAYA	1694/398	5	1.2	55.8	12.2	4.7	32.9
CHICKEN DOPIAZA WITH CUMIN ROAST POTATOES	1655/391	4.2	0.7	47	12	6.7	37
MEDITERRANEAN TUNA PASTA	1688/398	7.2	3.1	56	20	9.4	28
ROASTED VEGETABLE & HALLOUMI QUINOA	1569/373	8.5	3.2	51	22	9.7	17
BEEF KOFTA CURRY	846/201	5.4	2.2	12	7.9	3.1	24
PASTA ARRABBIATA	1505/356	2.6	0.4	65	12	7.3	13
CHICKEN, VEGETABLE & RICE BAKE	1573/374	11	2.8	43	3.7	3.5	25
VEGGIE SPAGHETTI BOLOGNESE	1646/386	2.8	0.6	74	23	13	19
CABBAGE ROLLS	1515/356	5.1	1.9	36	21	9.7	34

STEWS and SOUPS	ENERGY KJ/KCAL	FAT (G)	SATURATED FAT (G)	CARBS (G)	SUGAR (G)	FIBRE (G)	PROTEIN (G)
SOPA CRIOLLA	1315/313	9.3	2.7	28	8.7	5.9	25
BEEF & SWEET POTATO STEW	1456/345	5.7	2	40	20	7.6	28
CHERRY COLA PULLED PORK	1498/356	10	3.2	15	11	4.1	48
COQ AU VIN	1190/282	4.6	1.1	13	7.2	2.5	45
SPRING VEGETABLE SOUP	563/134	2.7	0.2	21	5.3	4.2	4.5

NUTRITIONAL INFO PER SERVING

STEWS and SOUPS Continued...	ENERGY KJ/KCAL	FAT (G)	SATURATED FAT (G)	CARBS (G)	SUGAR (G)	FIBRE (G)	PROTEIN (G)
GARLIC, CHICKEN & RICE SOUP	888/210	2	0.4	32	7.1	3.6	15
RAMEN BOWLS	1567/372	8.6	2	34	17	8.9	34
PORK CASSOULET	935/222	4.5	1.3	17	9.4	5.7	24

BAKES & ROASTS	ENERGY KJ/KCAL	FAT (G)	SATURATED FAT (G)	CARBS (G)	SUGAR (G)	FIBRE (G)	PROTEIN (G)
RATATOUILLE CHICKEN	952/224	2.7	0.7	11	8.9	4.5	39
HERB-CRUSTED LAMB	982/235	11	4.7	6.2	0.5	1.3	27
IMAM BAYILDI	486/116	2.2	0.4	16	13	5.4	3.8
LASAGNE BOWLS	1361/323	7.1	3.4	29	9.2	5	31
KEEMA PIE	1647/389	6.6	2.4	52.1	20.4	11.8	30.3
ZA'ATAR CHICKEN	1571/371	3	0.8	34	15	4.1	49
CREAMY VEGETABLE BAKE	1422/340	14	7.9	30	15	7.5	20
LEEK & BACON TARTIFLETTE	1471/349	9.1	4	38	7.5	5.8	26
SEAFOOD CRESPELLA	1555/370	13	4.5	35	13	6.1	23
LENTIL & ROOT VEGETABLE BAKE	1289/305	2.4	0.3	49	15	11	15
MOUSSAKA CANNELLONI	1516/358	10.5	4.5	29.4	26	12	36
PIRI PIRI ROAST CHICKEN	1228/294	17	4.8	1	0.6	0.8	32
SPINACH, FETA & POTATO BAKE	1290/306	5.2	2.6	47	3.8	5.9	14
ROOTS ROSTI	532/127	4.6	1.1	14	6.3	4.5	5.5
PASTITSIO	1696/400	7.5	3	53	19	7.8	32
STUFFED SQUASH	1423/339	7.4	3.6	48	24	14	13
WELSH RAREBIT POTATOES	1290/307	8.1	3.9	40	5	5.4	15

SNACKS, SIDES *and Sweet treats*	ENERGY KJ/KCAL	FAT (G)	SATURATED FAT (G)	CARBS (G)	SUGAR (G)	FIBRE (G)	PROTEIN (G)
BARBEQUE POTATO WEDGES	597/141	0.5	0.1	29	2.2	3.7	3.6
KATSU CHICKEN SCOTCH EGGS	1085/259	10	2.7	17	5.8	4.5	21
COLCANNON	533/126	0.5	0.1	25	3.3	4.3	3.4
KETCHUP TOMATOES	158/38	0.8	0.1	4.7	4	1.3	1.2
MAC & CHEESE BITES	161/38	1.5	0.5	4.3	0.5	0.5	1.9
CORONATION POTATO SALAD	833/197	0.6	0.1	40	4.7	3.1	6
FRENCH PEAS	455/108	3.1	0.5	7.3	3.9	3.1	11
CAULIFLOWER TOTS	687/164	3.9	1	22	5	5.1	8.9
LOADED CAULIFLOWER TRAY BAKE	708/168	1.7	0.3	28	18	6.9	7.9
GARLIC SCALLOPED POTATOES	748/176	0.5	0	37	1.9	4.3	4.4
LEMON & CORIANDER HUMMUS	340/80	0.6	0.1	13	1.8	1.7	4.8
VEGETABLE PARMESAN CHIPS	1157/276	11	6.1	28	14	8.3	13
BROCCOLI CHEESE	587/140	5.7	3	9.2	4.6	5.1	11
PINK APPLE SLAW	167/40	0.5	0	6.3	5.6	2.3	1
QUICKLES	195/46	1.1	0.1	5.8	4.7	1.8	2.2
ROASTED ROOT VEGETABLES WITH GARLIC & ROSEMARY	587/140	1.7	0.3	23	15	10	3.5
RUSSIAN SALAD	501/119	0.6	0.1	17	9.3	5.4	8.6
BATATAS PICANTES	929/220	1.6	0.3	42	15	5.7	4.7
PEACHES & CREAM FRENCH TOAST	959/229	6.9	1.8	19	6.1	3.7	19
RASPBERRY & ELDERFLOWER SWIRL	484/114	0.5	0.1	9.4	9.3	3.1	15
STRAWBERRY & PEACH ICE LOLLIES	39/9	0.5	0.1	1.4	1.4	0.7	0.5

ACCOMPANIMENTS	ENERGY KJ/KCAL	FAT (G)	SATURATED FAT (G)	CARBS (G)	SUGAR (G)	FIBRE (G)	PROTEIN (G)
BASMATI RICE (50G DRY/125G COOKED)	737/173	0.5	0.1	38	0	0.5	4.3
EGG NOODLES (1X38G NEST)	549/129	0.8	0.1	25	0.6	1.5	5
BAKED POTATO (ABOUT 170G)	695/164	0.5	0.2	34	2.3	4.3	4.1
BAKED SWEET POTATO (SMALL: ABOUT 135G)	520/123	0.5	0.1	27	7.4	2.9	1.6
BAKED SWEET POTATO (LARGE: ABOUT 238G)	920/217	0.7	0.2	48	13	5.1	2.8
MINI CORN ON THE COB (70G)	134/32	0.8	0.1	4.1	0.5	2.3	1.4
PASTA (50G DRY/100G COOKED)	739/174	0.8	0.1	35	1	1.9	6.2
MUSHY PEAS (¼ SERVING OF 300G TIN)	273/65	0.5	0.1	9.5	1.2	2.3	4.3
BAKED BEANS (¼ SERVING OF 420G TIN)	397/94	0.5	0.1	15	4.9	5.1	5.3
MIXED SALAD (75G)	64/15	0.5	0.1	1.5	1.1	0.9	1.1
STEAMED VEGETABLES (80G)	160/38	0.5	0.1	5	2.8	1.9	2.7
WHOLEMEAL BREAD ROLL (60G)	644/153	2	0.5	25	1.5	3.3	6.8
SEEDED WHOLEMEAL BREAD ROLL (60G)	773/184	4.9	0.8	25	2.1	4	7.9

INDEX

Page numbers in italics refer to images

ACKNOWLEDGEMENTS

Wow! A second book! None of this would have been possible without the help of so many fab people.

We want to say a huge thank you firstly, to all of our followers on social media and all those who continue to make our recipes and let us know what you want next! We're so proud that Pinch of Nom has helped, and continues to help, so many people.

Thank you to our publisher Carole, Martha, Bríd, Jodie and the rest of the team at Bluebird for helping us create this book and believing in Pinch of Nom enough for there to be a second book! Major thanks also to our agent Clare for your unwavering support and guidance.

To Mike for the ace photos and to Kate for making our food look so, so good. Big thanks go out to Emma for designing yet another incredible book.

We also want to thank our friends and family who have made this book possible. Special thanks go to Laura, Emma, Lisa and Meadows for the endless hours you've put into this and for working so hard to get things right! Additional thanks go to Vince, Sydney and Sophie. We're so, so proud to work with you lot.

To our wonderful moderators and online support team; thank you for all your hard work keeping the peace and for all your support.

Our thanks also to our amazing taste testing group again for all your help in sending your honest feedback and suggestions. We really appreciate the time you give to support us.

Ginger Cat, Freda and Brandi for the daily moments of joy. And finally … huge thanks go to Paul for your unwavering support. And to Cath who is never forgotten.

ABOUT THE AUTHORS

KATE *and* KAY

Founders of Pinch of Nom
www.pinchofnom.com

Kate Allinson and Kay Featherstone owned a restaurant together on the Wirral, where Kate was head chef. Together they created the Pinch of Nom blog with the aim of teaching people how to cook. They began sharing healthy, slimming recipes and today Pinch of Nom is the UK's most visited food blog with an active and engaged online community of over 1.5 million followers.

Keep on track with the new

**PINCH OF NOM
FOOD PLANNER:
EVERYDAY LIGHT**

PUBLISHING JUNE 2020

THANKS TO ALL THE PINCH OF NOM TASTE TESTERS

HANNAH DURANT

Shannon HARRIMAN

CHARLENE SHARMAN

NIAMH SHINE

LENA DENT

JAN LE...

LIZ LEVIS

LUCI VINŠOVÁ

EMMA ARNOLD

RACHEL HOARE

STEPHANIE CONNELLY

Mich... JACKS...

JULIE SWAYZE

Karen PEARSON

NATHAN WINFIELD

KATHRYN READ

LAURA CLIFFORDE

ANGE... HARRI...

Charles SWYER

Tara BROWN

Joanne HUDDART

JENNY DEVLIN

JULIA HARRIS

BEC... WRIG...

ALYSSA ANKRAH

BRIAN HOPCROFT

NATALIE LAVERY

PAULA GLASBEY

CAROLINE YORKE

CLAIRE

LAUREN NAPIER

JO LARDER

Nicole DEVLIN

Anita Sanderman

LYNN HARGREAVES -McCALLUM

AILE... O'TO...

JIM FORD

JUDITH HUNTER

Louise WRIGHT

KATRINA CANN

Sophie HUCKSTEP

MEGA... O'TO...

RIA TONGE

AMANDA CAMERON

KIRSTY SANDERSON

LORNA HENDERSON

KATY BROWN

BEVER... JOHNS...

Nicola MAYREN

Helen Pettit

KAROLYNNE BOLGER

DEIRDRE COOKE

LEYLA PATTISON

VICTO... PRIEST...

Niamh O'REGAN

Fiona SMALL

Lara RAWLINGS

Simone KELLY

JESSICA KINSON

LIND... HEDL...